'Back in 1988, two possibly 'wild-eyed' and optimistic Christian doctors with two young children went to serve with the Overseas Services Bureau (formerly known as Australian Volunteers Abroad) at Aitutaki in the southern Cook Islands.

'This very readable book is written in 33 short chapters (and an epilogue) centred around a theme or topic or incident. They are written as tales, not tall stories, about people met, faith challenged and deepened, and experience gained. Chapters abound with whimsical vignettes about local people and customs, and frequent cultural misunderstandings that often illustrated how much we all have in common.

'The tales illustrate a wonderful love and resonance with the local people, and some stories vividly illustrate the way they were able to cope with minimal medical technology and obtain necessary supplies. Mike even found time to preach while juggling cross-nation arrangements to enable an emergency medical evacuation.

'The most poignant personal reflection is found in 'Final Days', and it is worth obtaining the whole volume just to read this one chapter. The personal story illustrates their Christian faith in the context of the medical issues that they constantly grappled with, ultimately illuminating the whole message of serving and being with people in whatever the circumstances. This chapter, along with the epilogue are very suitable concluding reflections.

'I commend this book for its whimsical and gentle encouraging Christian message of service and love. In this time of chaos and anxiety, it will help people to reflect on our neighbours, Australia and our place in the world.'

–Peter Bentley, Past-President of the Australasian Religious Press Association, and editor or contributor to numerous Christian publications and magazines.

'We were volunteers in the Pacific at the same time that Michele and Mike Browne were volunteers in the Cook Islands and met them at one of the briefing sessions. *Beyond the Reef* is evocative of many of our own experiences and I am sure of many other health volunteers throughout Asia and the Pacific around that time. In this book, constructed from diaries and letters, Michele provides a catalogue of experiences and insights into not only the lives and culture of the small community in which they lived but also the challenges, suffering and adaptations they had to make in their personal and professional lives. Dr Rua said in 1989 "Your contributions (both) and sacrifices will remain as one difficult to forget or substitute." However I am sure that despite the contributions they made (including lives saved), the impacts on their own lives and those of their families may be even more enduring. The book provides an intimate window into all of it.'

– Mark Harris, Professor of General Practice and Executive Director of the Centre for Primary Health Care and Equity at UNSW.

'As human beings, we long to strike a balance between the familiar and the new, or the comforting and the exciting. We both crave the routine and security of home, but also wish to strike out and discover novelty with the power to take our breath away. Few of us live out there, though, in the wild unknown of foreign countries. Not many have the strength to be the only atoll of solid normalcy in a tumultuous ocean of strange.

'As an expat of now 14 years, I've felt keenly the strange way time begins to tick along while abroad, how every moment in the new place seems oversaturated with wonder and newness, and often horrible discomfort. While people back home seem stuck in the exact positions they were in when you left, you've changed in thousands of incalculable ways.

'The rich diversity and customs of island culture are on full display in Browne's experience on the island with two young children, including Christmas on Aitutaki, medical equipment dating back to the Korean war, massive islander feasts, and the hours of speeches that precede them. In these pages you'll have the unique opportunity to go aboard a cruise ship, a New Zealand Air Force flight, and SCUBA diving. Relive the sometimes harrowing, at times heartbreaking, and other times hilarious adventures in 'Beyond the Reef'. You'll be richer for it.'

–Brent Meske, author, and English Lecturer at the Joongbu University in Korea.

Beyond the Reef

A Medical Volunteer Sojourn

Michele Browne

AIA PUBLISHING

Beyond the Reef
Michele Browne
Copyright © 2020
Published by AIA Publishing, Australia
ABN: 32736122056
http://www.aiapublishing.com

All rights reserved. No part of this publication may be reproduced, stored in a retrieval system or transmitted in any form or by any means electronic, mechanical, audio, visual or otherwise, without prior permission of the copyright owner. Nor can it be circulated in any form of binding or cover other than that in which it is published and without similar conditions including this condition being imposed on the subsequent purchaser.

Paperback: ISBN: 978-1-922329-10-3

Cover design by K. Rose Kreative

Cover Image Captions:
Top: Beach scene on Aitutaki.
Middle: Aerial photograph of Aitutaki island and lagoon with motus. Used with the kind permission of Ewan Smith, Managing Director of Air Rarotonga Ltd via email on 4/6/2020.
Bottom: Motel where we had the Raro briefing. Note the unfenced pool behind us!

Rule of Thumb in Medicine*

Some people will get better no matter what you do.

Some people will die no matter what you do.

Always do your best –

And take every opportunity to make a difference.

* A summary of lessons learned in Aitutaki Hospital (1988-89)
but applicable in medical practice generally.
Dr Michele Browne, 2020.

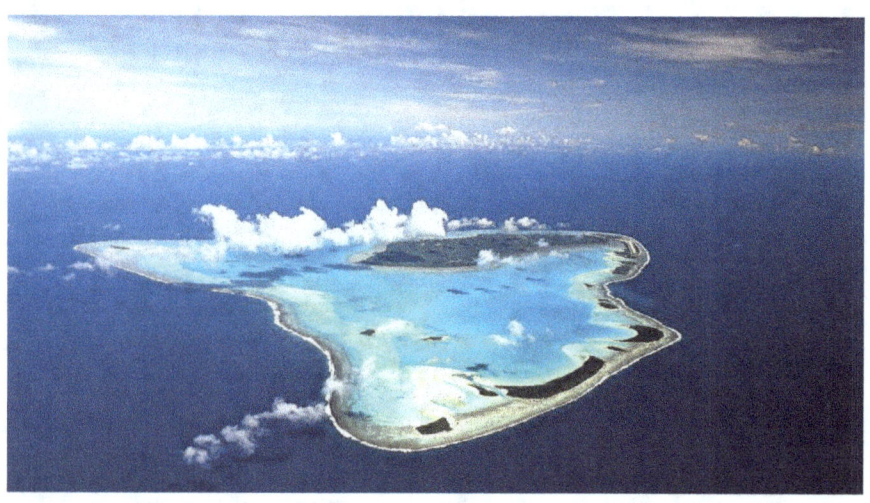

Aerial photograph of Aitutaki island and lagoon with motus. Used with the kind permission of Ewan Smith, Managing Director of Air Rarotonga Ltd via email on 4/6/2020

Contents

Introduction	1
Foreword	5
Acknowledgements	7
1 – Interview (Canberra – August, 1987)	10
2 – The Car	15
3 – The Fence	22
4 – Briefings in Brief	25
5 – Arrival	33
6 – Hospital Culture	41
7 – Hospital Community	50
8 – Papa'as and Places	60
9 – Visitors (Part I)	71
10 – Kaikais	81
11 – The Tutaka	88
12 – Different Deliveries	96
13 – Achievements and Amusements	108
14 - Supplies	119
15 – Mosquito Management	132

16 – Families	**138**
17 – Devious Devices	**150**
18 – Dangers and Delights	**162**
19 – Births and Breeches	**176**
20 – Blue Babies and Bluff	**186**
21 – Communication	**197**
22 – Solution B	**205**
23 – Christmas and Curious Conditions	**211**
24 – Ciguatera and Circumcisions	**220**
25 – Visitors (Part II)	**229**
26 – Fishing and Findings	**238**
27 – Repairs and Relief	**249**
28 – Veterinary Variety	**260**
29 – Incidents and Illnesses	**266**
30 – Visitors (Part III) Theirs and Ours	**278**
31 – Taxing Times	**285**
32 – Herculean Heroics	**289**
33 – Final Days	**300**
Epilogue	**310**
Christmas Card from Dr Rua – 28th December, 1989.	**316**
A Note from the Author	**317**
About the Author	**318**
Glossary of Māori Terms.	**319**
Glossary of Medical and Other Terms.	**322**
Timeline of Aitutaki Posting.	**338**

Introduction

I am not sure where the idea came from, but since our marriage in 1980, Michael and I had been keen to spend an extended period of time living and working in what was known at the time as a Third World country. As young doctors pursuing our General Practice or Family Medicine training, we thought it would be good for us to face unusual challenges early in our medical careers: broadening us professionally as we worked in a remote setting, learning to be self-reliant in a context of minimal resources, offering medical care to people who needed it more than many 'back home' and sharing skills with local health workers so that they could increasingly serve their own communities too.

From a personal standpoint, we wanted to develop friendships with others in this novel context, and anticipated that our western values would be challenged and our faith stretched by living in a culture that was very different from our own.

At least, that was the theory.

If you want to know how the reality worked out, you'll have to read the book!

We decided to explore a possible opening through the Overseas Services Bureau (OSB), an Australian non-government aid organisation (formerly known as Australian Volunteers Abroad) that matched 'volunteers' with requests from developing nations for professionals with specific skills. OSB assessed and interviewed us, and ultimately offered us a posting to the Cook Islands in the central South Pacific Ocean for 1988-89. We were sent to Aitutaki, one of the southern group atolls within the Cook Islands that had a population of about 2,300 residents at the time. The arrangement was such that we job-shared in one position at the very small local hospital, providing all medical care on the island with one other elderly local doctor. Since we had two very young children at that stage (Rhiannon was two-and-a-half and Thomas was seven months old when we left home), caring for them and assisting them to adjust to this new environment added to the complexity of our lives.

Now that our four 'kids' are young adults and beginning to have families of their own, we have a better understanding of why our relatives thought that we were insane to leave the familiarity, support and financial security of our Canberra existence at this stage of our lives.

'Why on earth would you take two small children to the middle of nowhere and put yourselves through so much, when you could just stay here?'

Good question.

We rationalised that if you want to have this kind of escapade, you need to do it early in life before the lure of safe, predictable and well-padded lifestyles becomes irresistible.

Following our arrival on the island, we recorded our adventures through erratic journaling and weekly hand-written letters home that our families faithfully saved for our return. These writings lay in a neglected folder for almost three decades, until a broken foot in 2017 and the ensuing immobility gave me cause to peruse them once again. It was interesting to immerse myself back into that era of our lives and I felt prompted to write about these unique and quirky incidents in the form of short tales, in order to record them for ourselves and any others who may be interested.

I've described our posting as a microcosm of Polynesian life at a specific point in their history and ours. My tales attempt to capture the coinciding of these two world views (ours and theirs), the individuals and incidents involved, and the impact that these events had on each one of us. All of the stories are true, although I've adopted some poetic license to give them more continuity, context and immediacy.

I've also included two glossaries: one of Māori words, and another of Medical and Other Terms, to enhance the fluency of the text, whilst providing explanations where appropriate. In order to protect the privacy of those I've written about, I've omitted or altered the names of most characters, unless I knew that they were willing to be named.

The book's title comes from a reference in one of my letters to my parents in December, 1988: *"Sometimes it seems as if life 'beyond the reef' is happening on another planet! We've grown very fond of this little island and its people. We've no doubt that this is the right place for us to be [in 1989]."*

This title denotes the reef as the boundary between life on the island and that of the outside world. I've used the phrase to describe us looking back from the outside world and the 21st century, 'beyond the reef' around the island into the Aitutaki community itself in the 1980s, and our unique experiences there. Conversely, the Epilogue relates both the profound changes we had undergone, and the adjustments we had to make, when we passed 'beyond the reef' and returned to our life in Australia at the end of our posting.

Regarding the Māori language: the term 'Māori' applies to both the singular and plural forms of this people group. Also, it is more appropriate to use the term 'Māori' to apply to Cook Islanders, to distinguish them from New Zealand Maori. Finally, while it is probably more respectful to use the term 'Cook islander' whenever I refer to the local people, I've abridged the term to 'islander' or 'local' to assist in the flow of the text. I hope I will be forgiven for any perceived disrespect – certainly none is intended, and I trust that my tales demonstrate the high regard in which we held, and continue to hold, the Māori people.

My hope is that, as you read these tales, you'll consider the particular challenges of living and working in a place so different from your own. Some of you may even be inspired to consider pursuing your own sojourn into another culture. But even if you don't, you will see how background and expectations are supremely important when connecting with others whose origins differ from your own – and the necessity of taking the time, sensitivity and humour to reach across divides to embrace others in our human family.

The year 2019 marked thirty years since we returned from our posting, so I felt it was an important milestone to acknowledge by finalising this small volume, although it also spilled over into 2020. If my writings have been able to convey a sense of this fascinating place in a brief fragment of time, then I have achieved my purpose in recording these stories – and even more so if they invoke an insight, a chuckle or a moment's reflection as you read.

I hope you enjoy our tales!
Michele Browne (2020).

Foreword

During July 1988, my wife Jan and I visited the Brownes in Aitutaki as part of a family holiday. While we were there, I saw the challenges that they faced when working in such a remote community.

At the time, I had envisaged that I could do volunteer locums in developing countries when I retired from medical practice as an Obstetrician and Gynaecologist in Canberra. But seeing the reality of what the Brownes had to face made me realise that this kind of work would be very different from what I had imagined. A specialist who works in a city hospital, with all the support staff that this setting provides, is in a very different situation from that which the Brownes had to face. Consequently, western doctors can lose the skills necessary for working in an isolated and minimally resourced setting.

The Brownes were young and resourceful and I witnessed this during our short stay. One case that particularly stood out for me was a schoolgirl who was run over by a bus and had severe injuries, including a compound fracture of her skull.

They managed this challenging case even though there were few supplies at their disposal, and very basic X-ray equipment on the island that had been left by a visiting dentist! Medical stock, even bandages and antibiotics, were in very short supply. Despite this, they were able to do a lot of good work for the Islanders, while also raising their young family.

This short narrative tells of their exciting and sometimes quite amusing adventures on Aitutaki. Michele has proven to be a good storyteller, and her faith and good humour also show through. Jan and I have enjoyed reading these tales – and we hope that you will do so too!

Dr Denis Appel
Canberra, ACT.
Australia.
January, 2018

Acknowledgements

My special thanks and warm gratitude go to my friend Peter Bentley, who initially edited my writing, completed a thorough review and gave me many helpful insights for which I am grateful. Tahlia Newland of AIA Publishing has provided invaluable editorial and professional assistance to make these tales more readable and interesting for a broader audience. Brent Meske, author and English lecturer has also given me substantial editorial feedback and support in my writing that I've greatly appreciated.

Chapter 17 is dedicated to Drs Denis and Jan Appel for their continuing involvement since their visit to Aitutaki to see us in July, 1988. They encouraged us as a family at the time, and particularly me with my writing more recently. We were especially grateful to Denis for his outrageously generous gift of a foetal sonicaid for Aitutaki Hospital – such a helpful device for our many obstetric patients and a remarkable reminder of two warm and wonderful human beings. Thank you so much!

Our thanks also go to Bonita, who was such a faithful friend to us during our time on Aitutaki, and has continued to be so ever since. The Stephens also stayed in contact until Rachel's untimely death in 1993, and Sam has continued his caring communications with us since that time. Thanks also to Dr Mark Hollands, whose record of the phone conversation that I've used in Chapter 21 is especially appreciated.

Thank you to all who visited us on the island – we really enjoyed connecting with each one of you, and you are listed in the Timeline at the end of the book. We especially thank our parents (Bruce & Marguerite Cole and Mac & Ena Browne) and my sister Marguerite Jones, her husband Philip and their four beautiful kids (Heidi, Ben, Sarah and Bronwyn), who made substantial sacrifices to come and immerse themselves into our lives and experiences on Aitutaki. Each of you made our time there extra-special! Thank you also to those faithful folk who prayed for us, and who sent letters and parcels to us – every single one was unbelievably precious when we felt so far from home.

Thank you to Felix, our Swiss friend, who visited us in October 1989 (see Chapter 33). He has made available his carefully catalogued photographs to contribute to my illustrations in this book. His friendship and practical assistance at a very difficult time will also remain very dear to us.

Of course, my husband Michael has been my most active supporter throughout our sojourn and my writings, and he has often assisted me with his memories, comments, encouraging remarks and witty insights, all of which have helped me to stay the course to the completion of this manuscript. All of our 'kids': Rhiannon, Thomas, Chloe and Evan, and their families, have also been inspirational and precious to us both in countless ways.

Most of all, my thanks and praise go to our Lord Jesus Christ, Who has sustained us so faithfully and has always been our Wonderful Counsellor and Prince of Peace.

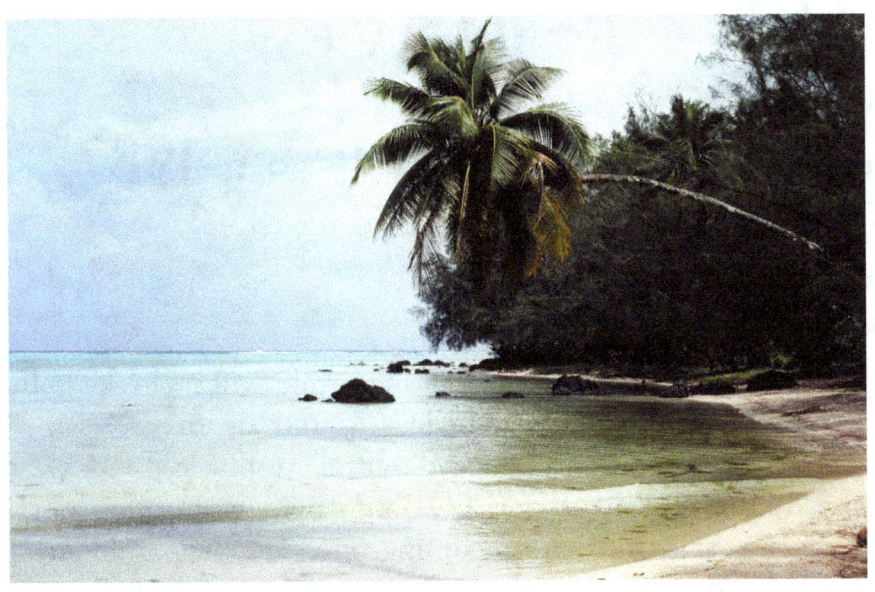

Beach scene on Aitutaki mainland.

1 – Interview
(Canberra – August, 1987)

I stared up at the austere building while Mike checked the address. A harsh wind howled around us in the wintry Canberra morning, and I hugged our infant son closer. We were already late, and the baby writhed unhappily with colic – not a promising start to the forthcoming interview that could affect our lives so profoundly for the next few years. Hauling pram and bulging nappy-bag along a maze of corridors, we finally found the appropriate counter where introductions were made.

After being ushered into the interview room, we sipped the kindly proffered Fairtrade tea while Anna flipped through various piles of paper. She was an earnest young woman who was dressed in colourful scarves, a cheesecloth skirt and jagged earrings that swung about wildly whenever she raised her head to focus on our answers.

We had come to the Overseas Services Bureau (formerly

known as Australian Volunteers Abroad) for an interview that was part of the process designed to connect Australian professionals with overseas requests for assistance. Since we were both doctors, our Plan was to work for 1988-89 in what was known at the time as a 'Third World' country, keenly anticipating that such roles would open up global perspectives and unique challenges for us early in our careers. We hoped to develop a broad range of practical, medical and life-skills and use them to benefit people who had less access to appropriate care compared with our compatriots. Our Plan was received with bewilderment by family and conflicting opinions from our peers, but we pushed ahead regardless, naïvely believing that such an adventure prior to having school-aged kids would somehow prove to be beneficial for us all.

Two slight complications at this stage were our two-year old daughter Rhiannon and three-month old son Thomas; but since they were both eminently portable, we saw them as no deterrent to the Plan progressing, although we had outsourced Rhiannon to friends for this morning's appointment.

The original paperwork had been complex, but served to forewarn us of the kinds of scenarios we might face in the ensuing interview. We had stayed up late the previous night to practise sensitive statements and pithy assertions that we hoped would convince OSB we were just what they were looking for, even though we didn't know exactly what that was. Anna's initial questions lulled us into a false sense of security: background statistics, our preferences for locations, what we had to offer and so forth. I kept Thomas quiet with his usual interminable breastfeeds, but these were followed by a progressive outflow of gas and liquid from the other end of his tiny but highly active intestinal tract.

The accompanying noises and odours made it hard to focus

on the increasingly complex questions that Anna engineered:

'What do you think about the concerns of de-skilling local people by your interventions?'

'How do you intend to connect with those who are very different culturally and linguistically from yourselves?'

'What legacy do you wish to leave behind in your designated country, before you return home to Australia?'

We took it in turns: one of us would answer as calmly and humbly as possible, whilst the other dropped to the floor, rifled through our gear, and repeatedly changed Thomas' nappy, or his entire outfit, depending on the extent of effluent involved.

The strain intensified as my mind darted around carefully nuanced responses, while Mike tried to be as spontaneous and sincere as possible. Knowing that we would be required to live in local housing on low-grade pay with minimal medical resources, it was important to appear to be as professional yet serene as possible, despite the escalating sense of angst that enveloped us.

Finally, Anna piped up with a critically important and apparently climactic question:

'Do you think it is necessary and desirable on a global scale for more wealthy nations to involve themselves in the affairs of their poorer neighbours, possibly causing more harm than good?'

We looked at each other in a state of near panic. *What was the right answer to that curly one?* Unable to read each other's distracted non-verbal cues, we hesitated for an uncomfortably long moment. Anna looked up and her earrings jangled alarmingly as she stared at us, intensely attuned to the unacceptable delay. We winced inwardly. It seemed that our destiny hung precipitously in the balance, and the answer could determine the future of our entire existence...

Then finally, at the same moment, we spoke with quiet

dignity and firmness:
'Yes.' (Mike)
'No.' (Me)

Anna looked from Mike to me: puzzled, dismayed. The pause felt catastrophic. We sensed our opportunity to sacrifice ourselves on the altar of foreign aid was being expelled with equal force to yet another pungent outflow from our young infant's intestine. Anna stared at the expanding yellow stain on our son's white jumpsuit and recoiled with distaste.

Running low by now on confidence, concentration and baby supplies, I plunged to the floor for a further change of outfit, while Mike scrambled to clarify our ambiguous response, gesticulating furiously with his hands to emphasise the sincerity of his words and distract attention from his stricken eyes.

'Of course, whilst understanding the need for commitment and sensitivity to the complexities of the culture we would be serving (whichever one that was going to be), we, as members of a wealthy nation, would be zealous Ambassadors of Australia, giving of ourselves tirelessly, generously, to strengthen the afflicted, support the weak – *without* leaving a single blemish on the integrity of the local society and its ageless traditions...'

The deep frown on Anna's brow eased slightly, she breathed more easily and nodded sagely at this entirely correct (albeit, impossibly meaningless) response. When she had finished jotting extensive notes on her pad of recycled paper, she sighed gently and bestowed a tiny smile of satisfaction on us both. It seemed to our unnerved instincts to say:

'You have done well, my children.'

It appeared the ordeal was nearing an end.

We gathered up the copious array of soiled linen into plastic bags and settled our infant, who was now finally asleep. We had exhausted our supply of pluckiness, passion and professionalism, exquisitely tempered by empathy, sensitivity and humanity, and felt as limp as the nappy-bag that I now hooked over the handles of the pram. Trying one last word of lightness to end the trial, I gave a small laugh and apologised for the constant diversion of attention from the interview.

Anna looked puzzled and frowned suspiciously: 'What do you mean?'

'Well, we needed to change Thomas four times, that's all. It must have been distracting for you…'

She smiled faintly, and with a gentle shake of her head, commented: 'No, I didn't notice that at all.'

I suppressed a huff of peevish irony. *So much for 'the overwhelming importance of observing sensitive nonverbal cues in challenging social encounters'*, I thought, reflecting on the advice we'd read the previous night about cross-cultural communications.

Rising from her chair, Anna navigated her way cautiously around us and the pram laden with plastic bags. She opened the door and turned back to us for her final benediction. With an expansive gesture of her hands, she solemnly announced:

'You'll be hearing from us in due course.'

2 – The Car

Miraculously, not only did we survive the interview, but we were surprised to discover that OSB had accepted us. After all, we only wanted to go to an obscure location for two years at a fraction of our usual salary, paying excessive local taxes and rent, foregoing all other financial entitlements, living under local conditions with no running hot water, to work 24/7 with minimal medical resources or back-up, and only radio telephone contact with the outside world. Was that too much to ask?

Our main stipulations were that we wouldn't go to a country that had endemic malaria (since our children were too young to take preventive treatment) and we would only perform the role of one doctor between the two of us, so that we could job-share and mind our own kids. We also preferred a placement that was part of our General Practice training scheme through the Royal Australian College of General Practitioners (RACGP). It seemed that OSB had found a place that matched our entire wish-list!

We were delighted to be offered a job for 1988-89 on a tiny atoll called Aitutaki in the Cook Islands. Searching for more information at our local library, we discovered that this island was located in the same longitude as Hawaii and the same latitude as Tahiti in the central South Pacific Ocean. The Cooks were made up of fifteen small islands divided into Northern and Southern groups that were spread over a vast distance of 1400 kms. Aitutaki was one of the eight Southern group islands, along with the main island of Rarotonga that was commonly shortened to 'Raro.' It seemed that most Māori lived in the Southern group, while the Northern islands were only sparsely populated or used for fishing, copra or pearl-shell trading.

Being on the eastern side of the International Date Line, the Cook Islands' time zone was twenty hours behind Australian Eastern Standard Time, but their medical resources (we were later to discover) were about thirty years behind Australian facilities of the same period: a state of affairs that was to prove quite confronting for us on many occasions.

The family who were occupying this role in 1986-87, the Vandermoezels, were also Australians of the same vintage as us. They had published some descriptions of their island life in the RACGP newsletter, and their experiences sounded intriguing. They wrote that Aitutaki was a one-hour plane flight from the main island of Rarotonga and was well known for its large and very beautiful lagoon. While the setting appeared to be laid back, with opportunities for snorkelling and boat trips in stunning surroundings, the medical role sounded far from idyllic. I was keen to discover resourceful ways of connecting with local people, but learning the language and working in such a remote location were daunting prospects indeed.

We corresponded by snail mail with the Vandermoezels during the latter part of 1987 and they passed on an abundance of practical information about what we could expect, both medically and socially, and how to best prepare for our stay.

Since they also had young children, their advice was especially relevant and provoked many intense discussions between Mike and me as we tried to project ourselves into this mysterious and somewhat paradoxical environment.

Sometimes we were barely game to ask each other why we had made this unlikely decision – after all, the answers proved elusive and we didn't want to sound as insane as many folk thought that we were.

Several months after our interview, when Mike arrived home from work, the kids were in their pyjamas and Rhiannon was pushing her baby brother around our small living room in his pram.

'Hello, you,' he said to Thomas and, tickling Rhiannon under her arm, he added: 'And you.'

'Hello you, too!' she shrieked, 'I went to the park today with my friend Ben.'

'Did you now?' Mike lifted Thomas out of the pram and put him into his high-chair.

'Yes,' she continued, 'And we played on the see-saw and the swing for *one whole hour*, didn't we Mum?'

'You sure did.'

I served out spaghetti and put a bowl of salad on the table while Mike lifted Rhiannon onto her seat.

'How's your day been?' Mike asked.

'Good thanks. Oh – and we got another letter from the Vandermoezels today.'

'Uh-huh. Any news?'

'Quite a bit actually. They've made a few surprising suggestions that are worth us considering.'

Mike gave a quizzical grin: 'Sounds intriguing.'

However, the conversation took another turn as the kids demanded our attention, so we deferred further discussions until later. Once they were settled for the night, Mike read the Vandermoezels' letter while I put on the kettle.

'Gosh, this is an interesting idea.' Mike looked up as I brought in the tea. 'I must admit I'd never have thought about bringing our own car with us.'

'Yes, I know, though it doesn't sound very politically correct, does it? We might just end up looking like rich westerners.'

Mike chuckled: 'Imagine what Anna from our interview would have to say about that, huh?'

'Mm, I can't really see her agreeing with it. But then she doesn't have to live on a remote Pacific island with two young kids,' I added with a frown.

'Good point. What they say makes sense though, doesn't it? I didn't realise that cars would be so expensive or hard to get hold of on the island or would rust so quickly. Bringing our own would mean that at least we'd *start* with a reliable car that wasn't rusted out.'

I nodded. '*They* wished they'd been able to ship over their own car, so they must think it would've made a big difference to them. Of course, since they came from Western Australia, it wasn't nearly as practical for them as it would be for us.'

'True. As they've mentioned, we'd have the advantage of packing it with extra gear – like toys for the kids, gardening tools and sewing stuff. Those things would be really useful when we got there.' Mike sipped his tea thoughtfully as he read further. 'And we could sell it at the end of our posting as well – so that's another bonus. I guess we could find out how long it'd take to ship one over before we make a final decision.'

I picked up some smocking that I was doing. 'And how much

it'd cost too, although it's bound to be cheaper than buying a car there.'

Mike nodded: 'I agree. Do you want to contact a few shipping companies tomorrow, so that we'll have some more definite information to go on?'

'Sure, will do.'

Further letters were exchanged with the Vandermoezels in which we expressed our concerns about turning up with an asset that most of the locals probably wouldn't own. But they urged us to ignore such triflings, pointing out that we weren't islanders (really?), we never would be, so there was no point in trying to act like we were.

We were deeply impressed.

Clearly, they had learned a thing or two during their time on the island. Maybe one day, we could be as wise as them…

Anyway, in the end, pragmatics won the day and we decided to ship over the better of our two cars, our Mitsubishi Galant called Hilda. Before she left, we proceeded to fill her to the gunnels — every crack and crevice including the wheel-bay shamelessly stuffed with the recommended paraphernalia, including indispensables like Vegemite and chocolate. If this was what we needed to do to remain independently mobile, mentally stable and emotionally intact, it was a very good decision.

My brothers then drove Hilda to the Sydney container terminal where she was stowed into the hold of the MV Norfolk Trader and transported to Auckland, Rarotonga and finally Aitutaki. At this time, we had no realisation that, with the various connections and weather patterns involved, this process could have taken up to six months to accomplish. We were also warned by well-meaning friends that, with so many car contents on open display, it was likely our possessions would be pilfered and the vehicle damaged or stolen.

In fact, on this occasion our naïvety was blessed. Hilda arrived in Rarotonga while we were still doing our two-week in-country briefing there and our reunion was sweet indeed. We then transferred her to the relevant freighter and witnessed her being unloaded from the tiny barge at Aitutaki harbour soon after our arrival on that island. There was a moment of gut-wrenching horror when she was being lifted by the rusty shore-side crane: swinging wildly in the air when suspended between barge and land, she threatened to slam against the wharf and shatter into pieces.

But thankfully, she arrived intact; and despite the predictions of theft and damage, the only loss we sustained was a broken pie-plate that I dropped during our enthusiastic unpacking at our new abode. In the total scheme of things, we considered it a very small price to pay.

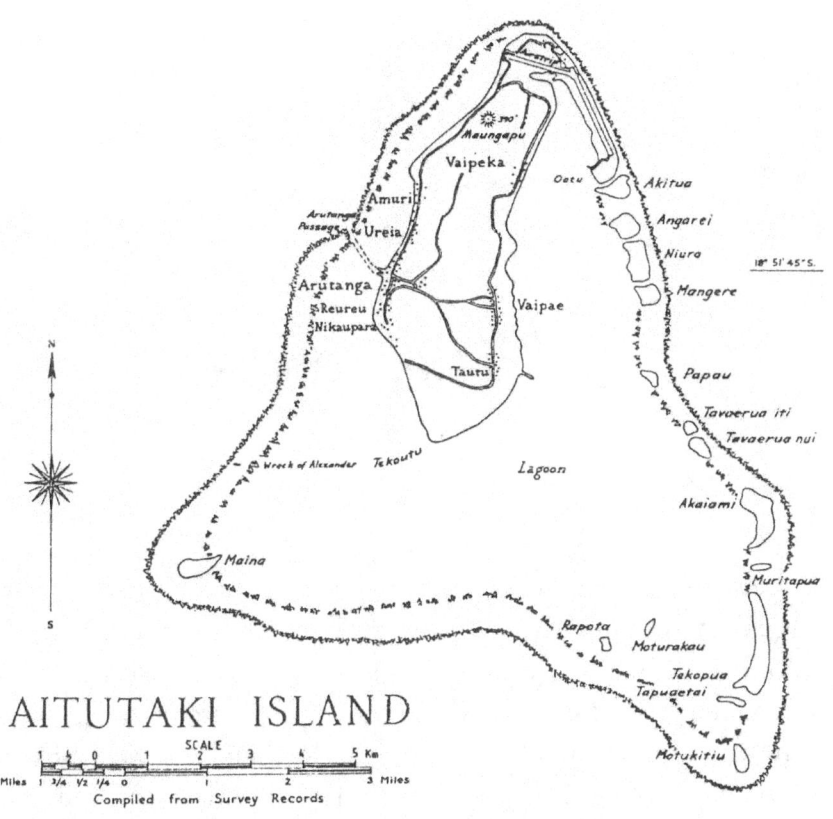

Map of Aitutaki island, villages and lagoon.
The fifteen lagoon motus (clockwise) are: Akitua (on which resort was located), Angarei, Niura, Mangere, Papau, Tavaerua iti, Tavaerua nui, Akaiami (which had a private house on it), Muritapua, Tekopua, Tapuaetai (One Foot Island), Motukitiu, Moturakau, Rapota, Maina.

3 – The Fence

It takes a great deal of preparation to leave home for two years. After sending the car ahead of us, there was still much to do. I look back on this period as one of immense stress and ambivalence. While we had some helpful information about Aitutaki through the Vandermoezels' feedback, it was difficult to project ourselves into the heat, isolation and work challenges that we were bound to face. Since most of our family and friends thought that our decision was absurd anyway, we couldn't discuss our anxieties with them; and Mike and I were usually too scared to talk about it with each other, since it was too late and humiliating to pull out now. So, we tried to look as stoic and carefree as possible, and that seemed to work fairly well for most of the time.

There were countless decisions to be made: what to take or leave behind, how to ensure bills would be paid, finding a tenant for our house and carers for our pot-plants, ensuring we had enough suitcases and so forth – all with the constant joys and demands of two very young children.

Mike responded to this ever-present uncertainty with a rather bizarre decision: to paint our back fence with Mission Brown Solarguard. Whether it was a primitive male activity to mark out his territory; an attempt to start at the edge of our lives and work ever inwards to find a core of existential meaning and purpose; or just a reaction to being overwhelmed with the great Cloud of Unknowing that had enveloped us, was never quite clear. No one had hitherto shown any interest at all in painting the Fence, despite its having been there for twenty years or so at this stage; and, being a corner block, the Fence was a very long one.

Whatever the rationale, the Fence became a big issue, and certainly a time-consuming one. Rhiannon wanted to play her part too, in her usual helpful way. Thankfully, she was still young enough to be satisfied with a beach-bucket of water and a small paint brush to add her own unique touches to the job at hand – a useful source of entertainment when she was in the right mood.

Family members came and went, boxes were packed and stored, cupboards emptied and suitcases filled, lists were written and ticked off – and paling by paling, the Fence neared completion. We went on a lengthy sojourn to bid farewell to folk from near and far, and did a two-week locum in a remote one-doctor town, where medical responsibilities included all of the obstetrics and DIY taking and developing of X-rays. This gave us a taste of just how little sleep you can get when you're on-call around the clock; and how essential a good sense of humour would prove to be. It was a rather sobering reality check, when we might otherwise have waxed lyrical (at least to everybody else) about the projected benefits of our two-year posting.

We gradually inched closer to our final Departure Day – the flight to Melbourne on 13th January, 1988 – for our Australian pre-departure briefing.

Our stress levels were climbing.

Even some Jehovah's Witnesses who appeared at our door to exhort us to follow their ways, realised we were far too distracted and tetchy to make their spiel worthwhile, and left us to trudge through our residual tasks in the hot, dry summer. The final days were a blur of trips to the rubbish dump, meals dropped off by friends, wiping out cupboards, and farewell events where we were showered with well-meaning gifts and cards.

Before falling into our own bed on that last weary night, beset by anxiety and mute with exhaustion, we stood on our back doorstep to contemplate the inexorable chain of events that we had set in motion. Praying silently for the times ahead, the inevitable challenges we would face, and the unknown as to whether or not we would survive them, we gazed upon one tiny piece of certainty:

The Fence was done.

4 – Briefings in Brief

The morning of our departure to Melbourne dawned and, as we went through our final checklist in the early hours, Mike was sitting at the kitchen bench with Rhiannon's backpack on his lap.

'I don't know,' Rhiannon shouted from her bedroom.

'You've got to figure out which one to take,' I called back, 'They're not going anywhere if we don't put them in.'

I turned to Mike. 'You'll still need to do one more trip to the dump before we go.'

Mike sighed. 'Yes, I know, but I'm trying to sort out Rhiannon's carry-on luggage.'

'Carry-on indeed,' I muttered fretfully.

Rhiannon padded into the living room that held five bulging rubbish bags, four open suitcases, and several other backpacks that still awaited their final contents. She appeared to be just as panicked as I felt, with her arms full of soft toys. My mind was almost obsessed with portability at this point and how to fit all the essentials into our limited luggage allowance. I scrambled to make a decision.

'How about Kev Koala?' I asked, nodding towards a toy in her left hand.

'You said they don't have gum trees over there – he'll starve to death!'

I looked at Mike with growing frustration. 'I'm… I'm sure Kev can eat, ah…'

Mike came to the rescue. 'Hibiscus – he can eat hibiscus.'

I nodded quickly. 'Yes – there's plenty of hibiscus on the island.'

Our two-year-old eyed us both warily, sizing up the possibility of an outright lie. In fairness, he was a hand puppet after all.

'Ok,' she said cautiously, picking up her backpack from Mike and putting Kev inside. She returned to her bedroom to replace the other toys in a cardboard box that was staying at our Canberra house.

'Thank goodness,' I murmured and got back to rearranging our packing with all the ingenuity I could muster.

Mike picked up the five bags of rubbish and the car keys. 'I'll do that dump trip now before we run out of time altogether. We need to be at the check-in by 9 a.m.'

'Sure, I'll hopefully have all this done by the time you get back.'

I sighed wearily. It already felt like a very long day and it was barely 7 a.m.

There was no time for sentimental reflections about leaving home in the chaos of getting to Canberra airport: the trip was executed at maximal speed, at least as much as our stately 1968 Austin 1800 could manage. Mike left the three of us at the drop-and-run area and parked in the long-stay carpark, where some friends were collecting it later that day. Pounding the tarmac back to us, he hummed the theme music from 'Chariots of Fire' as we rushed our baggage through check-in, and breathlessly made our way to the departure gates with barely thirty seconds to spare.

I sank gratefully into the plane seat and reflected that our adventure had finally begun. My thoughts flipped between anticipation and fear, but I was more excited than scared at this point – after all, we hadn't even left Australian shores yet!

The one-week OSB briefing was held at Janet Clarke Hall on the Melbourne University campus, with several hundred people in attendance. Most of them looked as naïve and altruistic as we did, although some were returned volunteers, who appeared far more sanguine than the rest of us. We met three other volunteers with their families who were also posted to various sites within the Cook Islands: one to Rarotonga (a draftsman), one to another remote Southern group island called Mauke (a teacher), and one (another teacher) who would live next door to us on Aitutaki.

We four families all left Melbourne for Rarotonga on the same flight on 21st January, 1988 at 4 p.m. and stopped in-transit at Auckland; but due to time zone changes, we arrived at 5:30 a.m. on the same date, which felt quite odd. We were disorientated with sleep deprivation as we stepped from the plane into the humid dawn, clutching crying children and damp luggage. Despite the time of day, we were moved by the greetings of local Australian volunteer families as they adorned us with floral necklaces *(eis)* made from Frangipani. Their unexpected and delightful welcome was especially heartening and helped us to build an immediate rapport with the expat community. Chirpy locals in bright shirts strummed guitars and sang islander ditties to welcome us to their shores. It was a lot to take in at such an early hour.

The other three families were whisked off to a local motel, but for some unknown reason, there was an error in the bookings *(promise of things to come...)* so we were driven to the uninhabited house that belonged to a relative of Ngu, the local woman who hosted our two-week in-country briefing. This was the first of many perplexing but character-building experiences, since we had no local language skills and were deposited by ourselves in a stranger's house for four days, with frequent inexplicable water stoppages and electrical blackouts to add to the other challenges. We had to collect buckets of water whenever the taps worked, to prepare for the numerous times when they didn't.

Being the wet season, between December and March, torrential showers were interspersed with bursts of bright steamy sunshine. On one occasion, there was a massive deluge lasting thirty hours that, at its heaviest, brought 300mm, or twelve inches, of rain in just two hours: it was quite spectacular even by local standards.

On Sundays, we attended the large and decorative Cook Islands Christian Church. The building was hot and the Māori services long, but the unaccompanied four-part singing was nothing short of a robust vocal triumph. Despite the language differences, we joined in with gusto.

On weekdays, we had talks each morning with Ngu that were followed later in the day by beach trips and meals in assorted venues. The volunteers who already resided in Raro kindly hosted a barbecue and cricket match on Australia Day, where we met up with more Aussie families, who were very friendly and gave us lots of useful local advice. They helped us to set up bank accounts and make arrangements with various shops to ship over bulk supplies of essentials like powdered milk and toilet paper to Aitutaki. We were very grateful for their practical assistance and ready hospitality – it certainly helped to counter the waves of homesickness and culture-shock that were already so disturbing and unpredictable.

Joining the other three volunteer families at their motel after four days provided us with company and strengthened our new friendships. Our daily informal meetings took place in an outside courtyard adjacent to a large unfenced swimming pool. This was rather disconcerting, since the four families included a total of seven children, whose ages ranged between seven months and five years. Ngu shared practical tips about basic language skills, customs and the subtleties of social etiquette in our new home.

One morning during her orientation talk, she advised us to give local politics a wide berth. She explained that, while Polynesians are generally laid back about many things, political feelings could run deep, and any discussion about such matters should be politely deflected with phrases such as: 'I respect the Government of the day.'

We were nodding in agreement with this advice when Mike suddenly jumped to his feet, dropped his coffee cup and pushed through our circle of chairs. Running frantically to the far side of the pool, he dived in fully clothed.

'What's he doing?' exclaimed a few incredulous bystanders.

We hurried across and were horrified to see the two-year-old daughter of one of the volunteer families floating perfectly still, with arms and legs outstretched, about a metre below the water's surface. Mike grabbed her quickly and dragged her to the edge of the pool where some others pulled her up onto the nearby grass.

'Is she OK?' a few voices said in hushed tones.

Feeling breathless with fear, I turned her onto her side and a mouthful of water flowed out. Thankfully, this was followed by a quick gasp and she began to howl. Many of the rest of us also joined in, weeping with relief that there was evidently no permanent harm done, while Mike hoisted himself out of the pool.

'How did you see her?' the traumatised mother asked.

'Just a flicker out of the corner of my eye,' Mike replied as he stood there, shivering and dripping; 'She didn't make a sound – it would've been so easy to miss her falling in altogether.'

We were all deeply shaken and the morning meeting abruptly concluded for the day. We found the setting somewhat fraught after that episode and took turns to watch the children more carefully during our remaining briefing sessions.

~

Being medical volunteers, our family had several trips to Rarotonga Hospital to meet various officials there. Like most islanders, they were fond of children, and plied ours with pawpaws and wedges of crunchy coconut *(uto)* to welcome us. The Minister for Health, the Director General of Health and one other doctor were Māori, and all of them had been medically trained in New Zealand.

Paradoxically, nearly all indigenous Cook Islanders who completed their medical studies ended up staying and working in New Zealand, where pay and conditions considerably exceeded those in their home islands. Consequently, most medical positions in the Cooks had to be filled by doctors from other countries, like us. The Rarotonga Hospital staff included a surgeon from Sri Lanka, a European cardiologist, an obstetrician from India, and a New Zealand Resident Medical Officer. Somewhat ironically, if they did return home to work, Māori doctors demonstrated that they were far more interested in the incentives of power, position and income than the rest of us by almost invariably becoming politicians.

As we were orientated to the health system, we discovered that Rarotonga Hospital was surprisingly well-supplied with basic medical resources. A wide range of medications, including sample packs from drug companies, but also imported stock from New Zealand, Australia, and further afield, were all available, along with dressings, and equipment for simple procedures and general surgery. More complex medical problems were generally dealt with by air-lifting patients directly to New Zealand.

Mike began an illuminating introduction to his medical work when doing half-days in the hospital's Emergency Department in the second week of our Raro briefing. It provided some curious insights into various Māori traits.

One sultry afternoon, time was passing slowly, so Mike flicked through an outdated paediatric journal in his cubicle at the far end of the Emergency ward. A strange plonk-scrape-plonk-scrape sound, accompanied by groans of pain, attracted his attention and he stood up and peered out of the doorway to see what was happening.

An islander was limping up the corridor towards him, dragging his left lower leg that was obviously fractured. This was surprising enough – but what was more remarkable was Mike's view of the nursing staff in the reception area behind the patient. They mimicked the suffering man and laughed uproariously at him as they leant against a row of wheelchairs, or used them to do doughnuts around him, in an atmosphere of wild hilarity.

Mike was astonished at this bizarre behaviour.

'Hey, how about you use one of those things to help this guy?' he called out indignantly.

The staff glared back at him, distinctly offended that this kill-joy was interrupting their fun. Then they all abruptly disappeared.

As Mike retrieved an abandoned wheelchair for him, the

Māori was bemused at this unexpected display of humanity.

'You stop their game, huh?' he said as he lowered himself into the wheelchair.

'Yes, apparently,' Mike replied, still shocked by the staff's response.

'They like a good laugh,' the man chuckled softly.

Mike shook his head, marvelling that even the patient seemed to see a comical side to this incident.

'So much for empathy,' Mike muttered to himself.

We later saw many examples of this curious attitude among the locals. Māori who showed signs of pain or distress were typically regarded with ridicule by their fellow islanders, even by those who worked in the 'caring professions.'

Girls almost universally had their first pregnancy in their mid-teens and generally went on to have numerous offspring. But if they exhibited even minor signs of discomfort during labour, the nurses shouted at them, or gave them a few sharp slaps for being unnecessarily attention-seeking.

Mike soon discovered that, if he prescribed analgesics for these young patients, the midwives responded with disparaging snorts and said something like: 'She's only having a baby – why would she need *those?*'

And suffice to say, unless he administered the medications himself, they were never given.

5 – Arrival

By 6th February, we had completed three weeks of briefings (one in Melbourne and two in Raro) and now eagerly boarded the twelve-seater Britten-Norman Islander plane for the one-hour flight from Rarotonga to Aitutaki. I vividly remember seeing the island coming into view for the first time: it was every bit as enchanting as we had been informed, with its narrow mainland fringed by a wide lacy coral reef that enclosed the vast turquoise lagoon. Apart from the main island, I counted fifteen other small islets within the lagoon, called *motus*. The whole place looked so appealing that we chatted excitedly about our plans to explore it in the months ahead.

The airstrip looked surprisingly large for such a small mainland. We later heard that it had been extended by the American military to enable the re-fuelling of bombers during the Second World War. As our plane approached the crunchy coral runway, my thoughts flickered between anxiety *(What on earth have we done?)* and relief *(Fantastic – we've arrived at last!).*

We were greeted by the hospital staff at the airport as they draped us in Frangipani garlands *(eis)* and floral crowns made from Gardenias *(Tiare Māori)* with their intoxicating scent. They hugged us enthusiastically and their generous smiles added to the warmth of their welcome. We piled onto one ambulance, a ute with wooden bench-seats on the back, while the staff climbed onto the other, and both traversed the coral-gravelled road to our new home to drop off our luggage.

The house was composed of concrete bricks, louvre windows and a corrugated iron roof. I was relieved to see that it was roomy and furnished with the basic essentials needed for our young family. The staff helped us to carry our bags inside and we complimented them on their cleaning efforts. I was touched to see that they had already placed pawpaws and watermelons in the tiny fridge – just right for our first island snacks.

I surveyed the scene with Thomas on my hip, seeing both the place as it was now and the work that still needed to be done. A tidal wave of fear and fatigue suddenly washed over me at the enormity of our decision.

We were finally here.

'I can't wait to have a cuppa,' I said as I turned to Mike.

'No, no – food first,' said the driver, and we were urged back onto the ambulance and ferried up the hill to the hospital. It was hard to get a good look at the place as we were quickly ushered out the back to the staffroom, where a hot meal had been prepared for us.

'Welcome to our *kaikai*,' the matron Kata proudly proclaimed, gesturing to the small feast. It all smelt lovely and we were keen to get started, but we paused to join in with the obligatory prayers and speeches on their side, and expressions of profound gratitude on ours. We were learning the drill after similar events at Raro in recent weeks.

It was very touching to be greeted by the rest of the friendly staff and the only other medic on the island, Dr Rua. I felt teary when meeting those with whom we would be working so closely, knowing that we'd need to handle all kinds of medical challenges together over the next two years. Most of all, we wanted to be accepted by our colleagues and the other islanders. After all, it was very clear that the Vandermoezels had been much loved and respected, and I hoped that we wouldn't prove to be too disappointing as their replacements.

We were quite hungry after our early morning flight, so the *kaikai* (feast) was much appreciated. Having been generously plied with chicken, potato salad, pawpaws and coconuts, the leftovers were wrapped in banana leaves and given to us in a woven pandanus *kete:* an ancient (but for us, new) kind of biodegradable basket. We appreciated the take-away food – not only because it was delicious, but it also provided easy meals for our first busy week on the island.

We were then delivered by an ambulance back to our house to begin the arduous task of unpacking. Between our farewell journeys within Australia and the two separate briefings in Melbourne and Raro, we had stayed in nineteen different locations during the previous four months. So it was definitely time to settle down at last, unpack our small treasures and make this place into our very own home in the Pacific.

Although we had seen photos of our island house that the Vandermoezels had sent, the sights and smells were quite unfamiliar. We had a few ceiling fans, but otherwise the sultry heat was very enervating and made it hard to unpack, especially during the long afternoons. Still, we wanted to establish a new normality as soon as possible, so this was a big motivator to get on with it – and even more so when our crammed car arrived on the island six days after we did. We enjoyed rediscovering our possessions once again: books, music tapes, family photos, the kids' toys and our favourite teapot were especially welcome!

The house had dining and lounge rooms, a kitchen, three bedrooms and a bathroom. We knew that there was a septic system and an inside toilet from the Vandermoezels' letters, but the old clay pipes were overgrown with vegetation and inclined to be unreliable, as we later discovered. The concrete floor in the living areas was covered with haphazard sheets of linoleum loosely abutting each other, in vivid black, green and red mismatching patterns that would have been popular in the 1950's. They were garish, worn and very grimy, but better than no covering at all – and added to the sense of the surreal that dominated our early weeks on the island.

While we steadily unpacked and looked for places to store our gear in the few available cupboards, the kids investigated this new setting for themselves. Since he was now mobile, eight-month-old Thomas quickly discovered that he could lift the edges of the lino and find millipedes and other small organisms slithering underneath. From time to time, when we heard him crunching during his exploratory crawls, we had to quickly extract these slimy creatures from his mouth before he swallowed them. Meanwhile, two-and-a half-year-old Rhiannon fearlessly tackled the gigantic cockroaches that scuttled around the house, and soon learned to smash them with her sandals or any other handy weapon. Children are so adaptable in new surroundings.

The bathroom layout was peculiar with a large permanently stained bath, concrete shower recess and separate flush toilet, but no basin of any kind. We made a mental note to add that to the list of things that we could raise with the appropriate authority at some point in the future. Since we had been forewarned that the house had no running hot water, we had brought over a camping shower with us: a large black plastic bag with a tap that we filled each day and lay in the sun – an early but clever innovation in solar heating technology. However, we foolishly omitted to bring a second one, so while the kids had warm baths each evening, we grown-ups had to make do with cold showers that were delightful in the summer, but rather less appealing in the cooler months.

The yard was spacious and included an outhouse that served as a laundry. It contained an ancient wringer washing machine that slumped dangerously against the side of a double concrete tub. I hadn't even seen such an appliance since my early childhood and thought that this species of labour-saving device was long since extinct. But it seemed that the Cook Islands were a handy repository for all kinds of expired products from New Zealand, and this was just another example. Nevertheless, with the daily collection of cloth nappies produced by our son, we were very grateful for any washing machine, even if it made hideous noises and was so rusted that it threatened to collapse without warning at any moment.

The kids were terrified of this prehistoric monster and wary of even entering the laundry, in case they never re-emerged. Consequently, my daily battles with the machine were solitary affairs, while the kids gave us both a wide berth. One of the upsides of this situation was that most days I had an hour to myself, but the downside was that hauling the lever to enable the wringer to work in different directions took so much effort and made such a racket, that reflective soliloquies were definitely out of the question.

The yard hosted a large water tank and many tropical plants: coconut palms; Frangipani, avocado, mango, pawpaw and custard-apple trees; and bushes of hibiscus and *rukau*, with edible leaves that were similar to baby spinach. We looked forward to planting a vegetable patch, and had packed seeds and gardening implements in the car to assist in this project, feeling confident that we'd soon be semi-self-sufficient in home-grown produce. The reality proved to be entirely different – but we had much to learn about this and many other things in the times ahead.

We had arranged with the Vandermoezels to buy their linen, curtains and day-to-day household articles before they left the island, and these were being stored for us. They had also posted us photos of the house and lists of the items themselves. However, as we unpacked, we noticed several curious anomalies.

'Hey Mike, I can't find the frying pan, saucepans or cooking bowls that are on the list; and there are at least six sheets, four pillows and a broom missing too. What do you think has happened?'

'Mm, right – and I don't suppose you've noticed the absence of the carport roof either, have you?' Mike replied; 'See, it's here in the photo.'

'Oh yes – so it is.'

We stared at the photo for a while, somewhat distracted by the kids rolling coconuts back and forth to each other across the lounge-room floor and shrieking gleefully as they crashed into the colourful cane furniture.

'What do we do now?' I asked, 'It's a bit embarrassing to ask the staff at the hospital – but maybe they'll know where things have ended up.'

Mike nodded, reluctant to raise this sensitive issue, but knowing that he had little choice.

He mentioned the situation to Dr Rua the next day at the Outpatient clinic and his colleague flushed with discomfort. As the morning rolled on, Mike overheard numerous intense Māori conversations between the staff as they quizzed each other about the lost items. Various phone calls were made and the ambulance drivers dispatched with their utes, apparently in pursuit of this salient quest.

Within a week, all the missing items magically re-appeared, and the hospital groundsmen reconstructed our carport roof with the galvanised iron sheets that had been recovered. This was followed by the attachment of four enormous stalks of bananas to the supporting beams – possibly an act of contrition on the part of the various anonymous borrowers.

'I want to thank everyone at the hospital for helping us out,' I said to Mike a few days later; 'It was so kind of them, and we couldn't have done it without their inside knowledge.'

'Sure, absolutely. But what do you think the usual Thank You gifts around here would be?'

We thought quietly for a few minutes, and then I said: 'Well I've noticed that food is always popular with the locals – it seems to be one of their major love languages, that's for sure.'

'Yes, like 99% of the world's population,' Mike added with a grin.

'Uh-huh. But I don't think that most of the locals would own ovens,' I added triumphantly, 'And that means *we* can make cakes and *they* can't. I think that *that* sort of food would be likely to go down very well, don't you?'

'Good thinking. Maybe we could take some to work on Friday for morning tea?'

We duly arrived with several trays of chocolate cakes shortly afterwards, and it was gratifying to see the delight on the faces of the staff as we expressed our thanks and ate large slabs together. In fact, we were relieved to note that, not only were these treats regarded by everyone present as deliciously acceptable, but it seemed that they were also considered to be culturally spot-on!

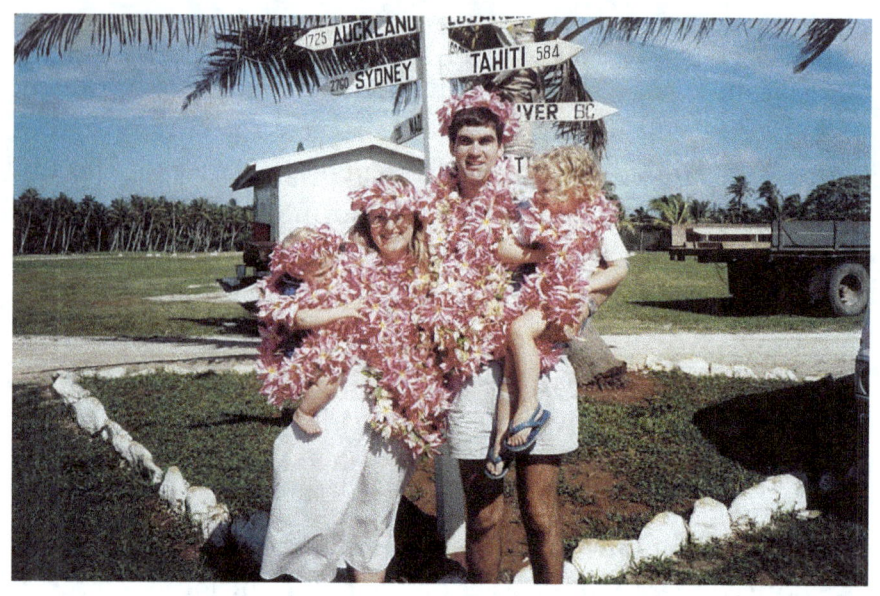

Our arrival on Aitutaki on 6/2/1988. *Eis* **provided by the hospital staff**

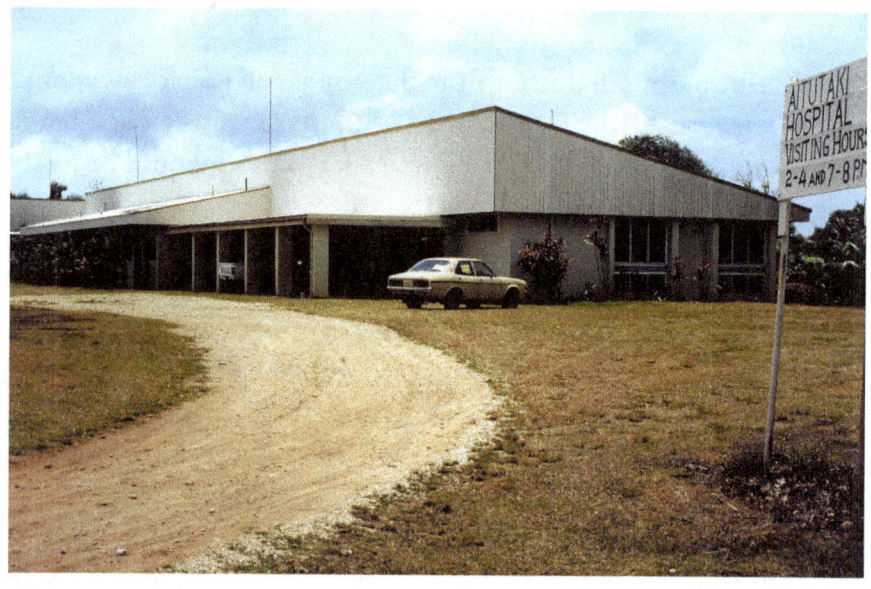

Our car (Hilda) parked beside Aitutaki Hospital.

6 – Hospital Culture

Aitutaki Hospital was located at the top of one of the few hills on the island. The views and breezes were enjoyable from here, but the downside (literally) was that our house was situated at the base of the same hill, and since most islanders drove gutless Honda 90 motorbikes with three or four people onboard, they struggled to get up the steep incline. Consequently, the locals generally defaulted to coming straight to our place. This resulted in numerous consultations taking place on our doorstep, which was far from medically or socially ideal for us.

However, since it would've been impossible for us to convey the message that we didn't want to be available at all hours to run an Outpatient clinic from our kitchen, we had to get used to these impromptu attendances and put up with the inevitable inconvenience. It certainly destroyed any semblance of boundaries that we may have previously maintained between our work and home life. In fact, it was the beginning of us understanding a little more of Māori ways: we discovered that cooperating with good grace and humour whenever possible seemed to be the best and only acceptable policy.

The hospital itself had twenty beds, a labour ward, operating theatre, dispensary, X-ray room and Outpatients department. The only other doctor on the island, Dr Rua, was a quietly-spoken elderly Māori, who had done his medical training many years earlier in Fiji. Apparently, he had tried to resign twice in the recent past, in order to spend more time with his wife, who often resided in New Zealand due to her poor health. However, he was repeatedly pressured into resuming work due to the lack of a replacement for him. He and Mike agreed to be flexible about the on-call roster, alternating every second night and weekend on-call, although this became 24/7 cover if either was on leave.

However, Dr Rua told us soon after we arrived that he was neither interested nor especially willing to do obstetrics. This meant that Mike supervised most of the deliveries and they formed a significant part of the after-hours load, whether he was technically 'on-call' or not. I didn't start work until some months after our arrival, since Thomas still demanded frequent breastfeeds and refused to be parted from me: we referred to him as the Original Velcro-boy!

From Monday to Friday, Mike and Dr Rua spent the mornings in Outpatients, where they saw up to twenty-five patients each. Following this, they worked alternate afternoons either seeing further outpatients or the in-patients in the ward. Mike took the opportunity of these quieter afternoons to check out supplies and equipment in various parts of the hospital. He discovered that the ancient Boyles' anaesthetic machine didn't work properly – a situation that seemed to worry no one but himself – so he stripped it down and rebuilt it. Of course, in a western hospital, only a qualified gas fitter would have touched the high-pressure reduction valves, yoked-pin index valves and flow meters, but with this kind of problem, if he didn't sort it out, it was highly unlikely that anybody else would. Versatility and resourcefulness were therefore useful assets.

There was an ante-natal clinic each week at the hospital run by the midwives. I was invited there to do a talk on breastfeeding at one stage, although rather ironically, I had to delay my presentation until I'd recovered from a rather nasty bout of mastitis, to permit a more enthusiastic version of my pep-talk!

Baby checks were conducted in the village halls by the Public Health nurses, who brought along a set of mobile weights that resembled grocery scales and babies were placed in the metal tray like small sacks of potatoes. These clinics were conducted with much merriment and camaraderie, as were so many things that the Māori did.

From time to time, overseas specialists visited Aitutaki to perform consultations or procedures at the hospital. Not only were they fairly ad hoc, but usually we were given little notice. One of these occurred soon after our arrival, when we received a telegram advising us that a New Zealander ophthalmologist and his team were arriving the following day. We were instructed that we needed to line up accommodation and support such as anaesthetics, medications and dressings.

'Right,' said Mike as he read the telegram to me in our kitchen, 'No need to give us too much warning then.'

'No, I don't think that forward planning is a particular feature of the Health Department here,' I added.

Mike frowned. 'Mm, so it would seem. Do you think you could ring around a few of the guest houses and see if they could take three extras for two nights and I'll check the dispensary to see if we've got enough dressings.'

'Sure, though hopefully they'll bring what they need in the way of local anaesthetics and eye drops. After all, they'll know what they prefer to use better than we do.'

'True,' Mike added as he headed back up to the hospital.

The following day, a Friday, the ambulance collected the visiting team from the airport while the hospital cooks prepared a small *kaikai* to welcome them. Floral necklaces *(eis)* had been hastily constructed by the staff overnight – it was unthinkable to receive guests without these essential elements of local culture.

'So, how do you want to run things?' Mike asked Dr Jeffrey, the eye specialist, as his wife Moira and an optometrist called Hamish tucked into the *kaikai* in the staffroom.

'Well, what we usually do is arrange for the Public Health team to round up as many of the school kids as possible who are aged between five and ten years, so that Hamish can check them out,' he said, 'And I'll see anyone that you know who's been complaining of eye symptoms.'

Things swung into action, and Outpatients was soon bustling with islanders waiting to be assessed. By 8 p.m. that evening, about a third of the kids had been checked, and the ophthalmologist had selected six patients who needed cataract surgery the following day.

'I hope you've brought your own local anaesthetics,' Mike advised the specialist, 'We don't have much of the sort you'd usually use in New Zealand.'

Dr Jeffrey laughed: 'Yes, I've noticed that on our previous visits. Actually, Moira has already packed them all and we've brought plenty of spare dressings too.'

Mike sighed with relief since our own stock was running low at this time.

The cataract surgery got underway early on Saturday morning. The clammy heat made them all sweaty under their theatre gowns, and the noisy overhead fans made little difference to their comfort levels. Mike did the anaesthetics while Moira assisted with her husband's surgery, having been a theatre nurse for many years.

As the list drew to a close, there was an unexpected screeching noise as one of the overhead fans suddenly jammed. The piercing crescendo sounded like a monstrous caged bird of prey.

'I think we'd better get this patient out of here,' said Mike, grabbing the trolley and running for the exit. 'Quick, Kata, turn off the fan switch, will you?'

Smoke began to billow into the theatre from the broken fan and flames ominously licked the ceiling. Coughing and retching, the other theatre occupants fled outside, while one of the ambulance drivers grabbed a fire extinguisher and sprayed vigorously. A groundsman turned on a hose and pulled it through the doorway to finally quell the flames.

The surgeon looked pale and shattered. 'We usually have a bit of fun with this outback work,' he said, 'But that's the first time we've had to evacuate for fire!'

'Well I'm glad that at least we'd finished the list,' Mike added, 'I don't think any of us would've wanted to go back there in a hurry.'

The team nodded in agreement, while the islanders laughed and chatted to each other outside – enjoying this extra dimension of excitement in their otherwise quiet lives.

Communication with patients proved to be very challenging, as many islanders spoke little English and we knew even less Māori. We found that we had to rapidly learn some useful medical phrases, and our mispronunciations were greeted with considerable amusement by the locals. It took us some time to realise just how economical they were with their use of language, even their own. Their alphabet comprised only thirteen letters, including eight consonants: G, K, M, N, P, R, T and V. (This explained why, with no 'L' in their alphabet, flower necklaces in the Cooks were called *'eis'*, and not the usual Polynesian *'leis'*.) Also, each consonant of Māori words is generally pronounced separately we discovered, and not slurred together as they can be in many English words.

In addition, despite the same spelling for some words, slight, almost inaudible, inflections could radically alter the meaning of words and result in substantial misunderstandings. For example, the word *'ika'* could mean 'fish', 'ocean' or 'vagina' depending on the way it was pronounced. The chances of getting it wrong were enormous and could lead to a social and professional mine-field.

There were further complexities around non-verbal communications too. For example, it took us quite some time to realise that a very slight, almost imperceptible, flicker of the eyebrows meant 'yes.' Not realising that a question had already been answered by this minimalist gesture, we would repeat our queries again and again, to the confusion and annoyance of locals, until we belatedly realised our *faux pas*.

Additionally, we soon discovered that the Māori considered it impolite to ask more than two or three questions at a time. This didn't allow much opportunity to get a medical history before being regarded as intrusive, rude or just plain thick. So between language subtleties and cultural taboos, the diagnostic process was very much abbreviated and required a good deal of guesswork.

With some locals who had virtually no use of English, Mike developed a wordless consultation technique that went something like this: An islander walked into the consulting room where doctor and patient greeted each other with a nod. Mike's questioning gesture was followed by the patient pulling up his shirt to reveal a skin rash. With another eyebrow flicker, Mike opened a drawer, pulled out a tube of antifungal or steroid skin cream and passed it to the patient, who nodded in acknowledgement. Mike mimed applying the cream to the relevant body part, with fingers and watch-pointing to indicate the number of times it needed to be used each day. After leaving the room, the islanders waiting outside, along with the patient, suddenly realised that not a word had been spoken on either side, and burst into laughter and enthusiastic applause!

It took us quite a while to adjust to the intriguing Māori attitude towards confidentiality and privacy, too. Islander houses were filled to overflowing with people (related or otherwise), all activities were done in pairs or groups, and it seemed anathema to do anything behind closed doors. Apparently, most locals spent their entire lives in the company of others and had negligible opportunities or desire for personal space. This concept was further reinforced for us when we hired a few high school girls to do some window-washing at our place a few months after our arrival. When they noticed that our kids slept in separate bedrooms, they were appalled, and made it clear they thought that we were being cruel to treat them in this horrifying way. After all, they pointed out, such solitary confinement would never have happened to them, or to any other Māori child in their experience.

These attitudes meant that medical consultations were conducted with the office door open, at the patient's insistence, while accompanying friends, family or others waited directly outside the clinic rooms on long wooden benches. Whenever patients were asked something, answers were often shouted out by those in the adjacent hallway, who shamelessly intruded on consultations with loud interjections or coarse laughter. This unscreened input became even more derisive if the patient had distressing or painful conditions, and we found it difficult to ask personal questions or give advice about sensitive issues.

On one occasion, I was consulting a woman in her twenties, who wanted advice about her weight. Like many Māori women, she'd had several pregnancies since her mid-teens with considerable weight gain each time, and she now measured a generous 160 kilograms or 360 pounds.

'So Mama Iti, you want to try to lose some weight, huh?'

There was a loud interruption from the corridor outside from someone with better than average English, but poorer than average manners: 'Yeah – you fat cow!' It was followed by raucous laughter from the small crowd listening in.

Trying to ignore this, I drew out a chart and calculated her Body Mass Index.

'Yes, well your BMI is 48,' I said, 'And a healthy level is about half of that.'

'You'll never get skinny the way you cram your mouth all the time,' was shouted through the doorway.

The patient and I paused to gather our thoughts.

'What do I need to do?' Mama Iti asked with quiet gravity.

'Shove your fist in your gob and leave it there!' was followed by more shrieks of malicious glee.

It was quite distracting, I'd have to say. I took a deep breath then discussed the idea of avoiding high fat/high carb foods with Mama Iti and wrote a list of healthy dietary options, while the invectives continued to flow in. I couldn't help thinking that many of those sitting outside on the bench-seats were of similar dimensions to the mama herself; but this seemed to be irrelevant, since she was the current patient and therefore the object of their insults.

We concluded the appointment with a few targets for the month ahead and the mama left with a calm nod. As she walked along the corridor on her way out, she gave a good dose of salty language to her commentators on the bench seats. I hadn't learnt enough Māori by then to know exactly what she'd said, but the intent of her assertions was unmistakable.

I knew that Mama Iti was related to one of the local bakers, so I recognised her outside his shop some weeks later, when I came to buy some bread. She had a thick cheesy roll in each hand and was enthusiastically tucking in.

'How's the diet going?' I ventured cautiously.

She looked at me with great excitement and said: 'Really good – I've already lost one kilogram.'

'Fantastic,' I replied, with growing enthusiasm; 'Only ninety-nine to go!'

We giggled conspiratorially and she continued her snack as I gave her a friendly wave and headed back home.

7 – Hospital Community

One quiet afternoon soon after our arrival, we took the kids up to the hospital to explore some ideas for improvements. The dispensary was very basic and often in a state of disarray, so we decided to start there, by cleaning it up and creating some order.

Mike picked up a broom and began to sweep the smelly rodent droppings from the floor, while Rhiannon found a flyswat and chased some cockroaches around the cupboards. I put Thomas in his pram and peeled him a small banana, then started wiping around the shelves with a damp cloth. As I did so, I noticed the bulky jars of medications and bottles of elixirs that we received from the Raro Hospital Pharmacy.

'It'd be really handy to be able to put tablets from these big containers into single-course packets to hand out to patients, don't you think?' I said to Mike when he had finished sweeping.

'Sure, and having some instructions on the outside in Māori would be good too,' he agreed.

We both looked around the small area, hoping for

inspiration. Giving a handful of pills to patients with a few verbal instructions seemed entirely inadequate, so we needed to find a more effective way to solve this problem. Our eyes hit upon some piles of old obstetric journals from the 1950's and I twigged to a possible idea.

'Maybe if we tear out single pages, we could fold them into envelopes,' I suggested and Mike nodded.

'And I think I've got a permanent marker pen in my room that we could use to write the instructions on the outside.'

'Can I help too?' Rhiannon piped up, having briefly run out of cockroaches to chase.

'Sure, it'll be good counting practice for you, love. I think I can see a pill-counter in this cupboard here.'

I stooped to check a low shelf and found a plastic device with a funnel that was designed specifically for this purpose. 'If you sit up here, you can help me to count out twenty tablets at a time.'

I lifted her onto the bench, washed her hands, then poured some capsules into a kidney dish. Mike began tearing out the journal pages, folding and stapling them so that nothing could spill out and writing the instructions in Māori on each one. I helped Rhiannon with the pill counting and pouring them into envelopes before stapling them shut. We started with antibiotics and then went onto courses of antihypertensives and other common medications to facilitate our consultations for the coming weeks.

We got into the habit of putting together further 'kits' every month or so and it became a family ritual on quiet afternoons. Some Australian friends later posted over small plastic containers into which we could decant elixirs such as cough syrup or liquid Paracetamol, and then affix Māori instructions with sticky tape. It was quite satisfying to solve these small challenges with whatever resources came to hand.

One afternoon, when Mike went to clean up the hospital's operating theatre, he passed the scrub-sinks where he startled the matron, Kata and a bevy of nursing staff, who were stripped to their voluminous white underwear. They were pummelling their families' weekly washing in the deep stainless-steel sinks in the hot running water. The tiled room rang out with cheerful chatter and peals of laughter, while the spicy tang of Lifebuoy soap floated through the doorway.

His arrival was met with loud shrieks, as soapy forearms were demurely clutched across the numerous ample bosoms. Stammering an apology, he averted his gaze and made a speedy exit. It seemed that the staff had learned the art of using whatever was available to maximal benefit too!

~

We gradually discovered that our workmates at the hospital had widely disparate education and training levels for their roles. Some of the nursing staff had done their qualifications in New Zealand and were reasonably competent. But others had not, and were often overwhelmed by embarrassment (the Māori term was 'akama') when asked about patient care.

One lunchtime, I came home from working at the Outpatients clinic and said to Mike: 'It's really strange, you know. One of the nurses called Tua always gives me the same blood pressure reading, no matter how many different patients I ask her to check. It's weird.'

'Ah – does that happen to be 130/70?' Mike asked with a knowing smile.

'Mm,' I nodded, 'Sound familiar?'

'Yes, she always gives me that reading for my patients too.'

A few hours earlier, someone had dropped in some parrotfish for us and Mike was cleaning and filleting them. I started to peel some *kumara* to accompany them for dinner.

'I guess we both know what that means,' I said thoughtfully, 'She doesn't actually know how to do BPs, and it's easier for her to give us an answer that sounds ok than to learn how to do them herself.'

'Yep – that's about right.'

'It's tricky, though isn't it?' I said, feeling dissatisfied with ignoring the issue; 'I'd much rather show her how to do them and get her to practise with me.'

'Yes, but that would mean making it clear that she doesn't know what she's doing, and we both know how badly that'd go down. Once the other staff noticed, her life wouldn't be worth living.'

I sighed heavily – he was absolutely right. We had already observed that any implication that someone was deficient in their role could result in a humiliating verbal attack from their work colleagues. Reputations were highly valued in this community and could be irreparably damaged by critical statements from those who were considered to have greater authority or status.

A loud crash sounded from the lounge-room and we went to investigate. Thomas had been trying to climb onto a large tricycle and both had fallen over. He was upset for a few minutes, but was soon distracted with his trolley of wooden bricks. Rhiannon ignored us all and went on with a cardboard construction she was making on the dining room table.

'I guess we'll have to let it go,' Mike concluded as we cleaned up the sink, 'It's going to cause more harm than good to bring it up with her.'

I reluctantly agreed. Then I remembered a short scenario that had happened about a week earlier.

'Do you know Tiare – that lovely girl who's one of the hospital cleaners? She and I have got to know each other lately, because she's spent a few years in New Zealand, so her English is really good.'

Mike nodded: 'Yes, I think I know her.'

He began to peel a pawpaw to have with lunch.

'She came up to me at the hospital last week and she had a big smile on her face. Actually, that was when I noticed that she was wearing a new white uniform, instead of her usual light-blue cleaners' one.'

'Ah-huh,' Mike nodded as he chopped the fruit.

'Well, she said to me: "Kata said they needed some more nurses, so I could be a nurse now." She looked so excited, but I just couldn't believe it.' I shook my head in amazement.

'Right,' Mike said, holding the knife absently as he processed my comments; 'So – all it takes to increase the number of nurses at the hospital is to hand out a few more white uniforms to the other employees, huh?'

I winced. 'Yes, apparently. If only it were that simple.'

'Mm, but it does explain a lot, doesn't it?' Mike added as he resumed his chopping.

'Yes, like the lack of even basic nursing competence.'

'Exactly – but sadly, there's absolutely nothing we can do about it – apart from trying to show *everyone* what we're doing when we do blood pressures and so on. Hopefully that way, those who need to will have at least some chance of picking up some nursing skills.'

I reluctantly nodded in agreement as I poured some glasses of water to have with lunch.

There was another crash from the lounge-room and we both went to check out the fresh cries of dismay.

The pathology technician, who was renowned for his potent home-brew liquor, was AWOL for much of the time – possibly fishing or drinking, we surmised. We became rather suspicious of his competence also, after noticing that whenever he was intoxicated (a frequent occurrence), he reported every Blood Sugar Level as 6.3mmol/l and every Haemoglobin as 120g/l. It seemed unlikely that so many random readings over two years would happen to be identical. But hey – who knows? Not him, apparently – and consequently, not us.

However, his unique skill-set came in handy on various occasions when we had patients with life-threatening blood loss, usually due to trauma or obstetric complications. He appeared to have an intrinsic knowledge of the blood group of every family on the island. Once he had checked a patient's blood group, he would name the appropriate donors, and an ambulance would be sent to collect them. The 'volunteers' would then be co-opted into providing direct donor-to-patient blood transfusions. It was a vital resource, since there was no way of safely storing donated blood on the island at the time.

Even in that era, we were aghast that there seemed to be only the most basic cross-matching procedures for blood types, and no checking at all for blood-borne infections. With a known 25% carrier rate of Hepatitis B among the Māori, the risk of transmitting this serious disease by transfusions was unthinkably high. At this time, it was also in the pre-HIV screening era – at least in the Cook Islands – so later on, we became even more concerned to consider the possible transmission of AIDS by this means. But when patients were haemorrhaging severely, we didn't feel we had much choice, and transfusing them in this way was better than their possible untimely demise from critical blood loss.

On one notable occasion, Mike needed an urgent transfusion for an obstetric patient with a serious postpartum bleed. The lab technician was too drunk to answer the phone and an ambulance was dispatched to drive him in. Mike collected the patient's blood himself, since the technician couldn't insert the needle steadily enough at the time. However, the staff member *was* able to do the blood group testing and soon announced two suitable donors. Once again, the ambulance drivers headed off to round them up.

The first proved to be cooperative enough, but the second had to be carried in from a local bar, where he'd been enjoying a big night out for several hours. Mike could smell pungent waves of alcohol on the breath of both the technician and the donor from several metres away. He was concerned about giving such a high dose of blood alcohol to the seriously ill patient, as there was at least a theoretical risk that it could cause uterine relaxation and thereby further heavy vaginal bleeding.

But time and appropriate donors were running short at this Friday late-night hour, so he felt he had to go ahead. The mama dropped into a profound sleep soon after the second transfusion, but there didn't appear to be any untoward side-effects. Thankfully, her bleeding subsided appreciably and she awoke the following morning feeling remarkably refreshed!

~

The Public Health Department was located in the hospital grounds and included three male officers and two female nurses in a single open-plan office. I was visiting Pua, one of the Public Health nurses there one sultry afternoon several months after our arrival. I wanted to discuss possible part-time work I could do, when I saw the system of contraception supply in operation.

Several local women entered the office and honed in on the nurses' desks.

'Hey Pua,' one of the women said, 'We need some more pills.'

Moana, one of the male officers called out loudly: 'No way, Pua. You know their men will be angry. They shouldn't be using pills if the men don't come with their women.'

He was clearly quite agitated and the other male officers made lewd gestures as well. The women huddled closely around Pua, who snorted derisively at the men. She cut a big figure – in both body and personality – and was not easily intimidated by a few aggressive males.

Rummaging through the contents of her desk drawer, she pulled out a handful of pill-packs of different brands and dosages. 'Here, take those – they should last a few months.'

I thought I should speak up from the side-lines. 'Don't you think you should ask them what they're already on and whether they're breast-feeding or not? Some of those packs might be mini-pills or high-dose pills and it's not good to mix them up.'

Pua shrugged her shoulders dismissively and the women scuttled out to escape the continuing jeers of the male officers. I was taken aback at this random and indiscreet way of dispensing contraceptives, but it gave me an idea.

'Actually, Pua – maybe I could run a women's health clinic in Outpatients one afternoon each week. That way, the mamas could get their pills and have regular check-ups too.'

Pua nodded slowly: 'Yeah, maybe.'

I was pleased to find a role that I could do that would hopefully make a difference to the local women, as well as being able to encourage the Public Health nurses to learn some new skills themselves. Maybe, they would even keep the clinic going after I left the island and it could be an important longer term legacy. My thoughts ran ahead with exciting prospects...

To her credit, Pua was supportive of the idea and helped to get the message out to the local women over the next few weeks. Most of them had never heard of, let alone ever had, a Pap smear so they were understandably suspicious of the process. Despite their objections, I insisted on seeing one woman at a time *with the door closed* to take a history, while Pua translated. We then did breast and blood pressure checks and I taught the nurses how to do Pap smears. In her usual manner, Pua ensured patient compliance by shouting loudly and slapping the women, but I persuaded her that, although a collaborative approach could take a little longer, it was more likely to ensure better cooperation in the long run.

Happily, this did indeed prove to be the case, and the Monday afternoon clinic became a very popular meeting place for the local mamas quite quickly.

~

The hospital gardeners were huge, athletic men who often wore a colourful hibiscus incongruously peeping out from behind one ear. Although they spoke little English, they were always tolerant and good-natured whenever we asked for their help. They also seemed to be the go-to staff members for any tasks that required extra man-power.

One afternoon, after finishing up her role in the dispensary, Rhiannon conned several of them into tying pink ribbons around toilet rolls for her, as part of her latest creation. She then rewarded them with a lengthy display of her new shell collection, rambling on about the minute features of each particular variety. Although they had no idea of what she was talking about, they smiled at her demurely, and seemed patiently and politely impressed.

~

We noticed that there was one time each day when the usual hierarchy of work roles seemed to melt into oblivion. Once the morning's outpatients were dealt with and lunch was had, there tended to be a single priority amongst everyone present in the hospital. In fact, it became difficult to distinguish the actual in-patients from anyone else at this time of day.

This was because a wander through the medical ward between 1 – 3 p.m. often revealed the entire staff: ambulance drivers, nurses, cleaners and groundsmen, horizontal on every available spare bed, impervious to all but the most insistent demands, as they lay snoring and snuffling alongside each other, and peacefully sound asleep.

8 – Papa'as and Places

Over the roar of torrential rain on our metal roof and fretful calls from the kids, I heard a knock at the kitchen door. I opened it and, to my relief, found two of our best friends on the island standing there, rather than another patient bypassing the hospital. Bonita and Father Luke usually came over on Tuesday evenings for tea and fellowship, and I loved their humorous stories and the next instalments of their gritty island sagas.

Our first months on Aitutaki had been clouded by homesickness, disorientation and cultural drift. Since everyone we met was a stranger, and many of them had very little in common with us, engaging with people often felt exhausting. I struggled with an erratic sense of ambivalence about even being on the island. Mostly, I felt bold enough to connect with those who lived nearby or we met through work, but there were other times when I found it difficult to leave the house at all due to overpowering ennui. The whole experience was certainly much harder than I had expected, and my emotions were often brittle and raw. Consequently, our friendships with these two were indispensable sanity savers.

Bonita, a delightful woman of our age, had been on Aitutaki for a year already, during which time she had taught Maths at the High School and become good friends with our predecessors, the Vandermoezels. Father Luke was a muscular and erudite Catholic priest in his early thirties, who had arrived on the island about the same time as us.

Mike made supper and we settled onto the lounge-room couches.

With mug in hand, Bonita began in her soft American accent, 'I've gotta get off this rock.'

Well aware of her issues, I smiled warmly. She dropped over to our place for a cuppa and mutual debrief after most school days, and our full and frank discussions provided an essential outlet for our many low-key concerns. It was so good to have her sharing in these daily dramas, no matter how trivial: we could roll our eyes, shake heads or chuckle together and help to restore each other's sense of humour and perspective – an absolute must, if we were to survive the two year posting with our mental health intact.

'This coral burp is doing my head in,' she continued; 'We found out today that the school principal still hasn't even *applied* to replace the two teachers that left last year, even though I've now got *forty-two* kids in my classes. If he doesn't do something soon, I'm gonna go reef-crazy.'

Luke's Hawaiian descent made him look like an islander, but he found the locals and their paradoxical priorities just as testing as we did. In his priestly role, he anguished over various ecclesiastical difficulties, and he followed on with his own tale of woe: 'You won't believe what happened to me this week: the congregation has decided that I have to supervise the flower arrangements *and* the communion purchases, as if I haven't got enough stuff to do already.' He shrugged his athletic shoulders in frustration.

As the heavy rain intensified, we shuffled our chairs closer together till our knees collided, not wanting to miss a single delicious word...

~

Cook Islanders conveniently divide the world's population into two discrete but extremely unequal parts: Māori (them) and *Papa'as* (us and every other non-Māori on the planet). There were only about twenty *papa'as* on Aitutaki, so we were quite diluted by the rest of the population of 2,300 people. As with many other remote non-western locations, the *papa'as* could be categorised loosely as: mercenaries, missionaries or misfits. (We probably fitted mid-way between the latter two.) Even among the expats therefore, there was a great diversity of backgrounds and reasons for being on the island. Consequently, while it was good to connect with them, the common ground between us could be very narrow indeed.

Many *papa'as* were men with islander partners and children, thus giving them access to long-stay residency visas. We gradually met many of them during the course of our posting, and became friends with those whose interests overlapped with our own.

One Saturday morning several months after our arrival, we drove into town to see what produce was on offer. The commercial hub in Arutanga village consisted of two small grocery shops, a bakery, the post office and a few other nondescript buildings. We walked into one of the general stores and stared at the mostly empty shelves. We were told that the last supply ship had been able to unload very little of its cargo due to rough weather, so the store lacked many of the most basic provisions, while the prices were remarkably high.

'I just wish we could buy some fruit and veggies,' I said to Mike, who looked exhausted after a difficult delivery that had taken up much of the previous night. He nodded disconsolately as we looked for some other staples.

'Are there any corn flakes, Mum?' Rhiannon asked, 'I don't want to have the same breakfast every day.'

I looked for cereals, but found none, and probably wouldn't for another month at least.

'Sorry love, we'll have to make do with bread or fruit. Maybe we could pick some bananas or pawpaws when we get home, do you think?'

She responded with a sour look, clearly not keen on that idea at all. The humidity made us all rather low-spirited and I wondered whether another beach trip would be preferable instead. Fortunately though, I found some tinned fish and dried soup mixes – they would be helpful for some simple meals, I thought. We bought a few things, then walked outside. We were about to get into the car when a tourist couple wandered up to us.

'Do you know how we can arrange a boat tour?' the woman asked hopefully, 'We've heard the lagoon here is the best in the whole country and we've come over from Raro for a day-trip to see it. But there's no sign of any rides for tourists.'

We looked sympathetically at the young couple.

'Yes, I know – it's not easy to find anyone who organises outings regularly,' I replied, 'Hop into the car and we'll see if we can find someone who's available.'

They responded with grateful smiles and clambered into Hilda, making it rather crowded with the six of us in our small sedan. The kids eyed them warily as we chatted about where they'd come from – Canada apparently – and they told us enthusiastically about how lucky we were to live on such an idyllic island. I cast an eye over the kids' grouchy expressions, our scant over-priced groceries and Mike, as he stifled a weary yawn, and gave them an unconvincing smile.

Yeah – it's absolute paradise...

We drove to Brian's set-up along the main road. The Aussie had run a wind-surfing and catamaran business for about five years, although the term 'business' was quite an over-statement. What really happened was that he sailed on the lagoon by himself, and if someone happened to find him just before he was going out, they could tag along too. During our time on Aitutaki, most 'tourist operators' couldn't be bothered to advertise themselves or to cater for *papa'a* visitors – it simply didn't suit their western escapism or laid-back island lifestyles. The most they managed was a tacky hand-painted sign at the side of the road, but no regular schedules. Brian was nowhere to be found, so we drove further along the road and slowed down outside Ned's house.

The Kiwi had previously been a commercial diver as part of a larger organisation based in New Zealand. However, for several decades since then, he had run his own scuba and snorkel business on Aitutaki, taking tourists out in his motorboat to explore the *motus* in the lagoon or to dive outside the reef. He had a local wife and a young daughter and was a pleasant easy-going fellow. But as we looked up his driveway, it seemed that no one was around at his place either.

As we drove along further, we came across one of the younger *papa'as* called Grant, a thirty-year-old Australian who had lived in the Cooks for about ten years and styled himself as 'more Māori than the Māori.' Whenever he could, he regaled Mike with stories of how to catch fish and local women – and seemed to consider himself as an expert in both – despite (or because of) having an islander partner and four young sons of his own. Mike drove up beside him and spoke through the open car window.

'Hey Grant, are you going out in your boat today?'

The 'Māori *papa'a*' eyed our full car, especially the tourists, and shook his head regretfully.

'Sorry, the wife's put her foot down, and I've got to look after my boys today.'

Mm – maybe he didn't live in utopia either, I thought...

The Canadians laughed at his despondent sigh, and we took a turn-off further down the road.

'Let's try Warren,' Mike said, 'He owns a guest house and is married to a local lady.'

He was in the front yard when we arrived at his place, so we introduced him to the Canadians and he agreed to take them out in his boat, along with some of his own guests. The day-trippers climbed out of the car and thanked us warmly, as we exchanged farewell waves. Warren wandered around to the driver's side for a quiet chat.

'I was wondering if we might be able to help each other out,' he began.

'Sure, if we can,' Mike replied.

'Maybe I could borrow your car sometimes to take my guests back and forth to the airport, and I'd be happy to give your family some lagoon trips in my motor boat instead of payment – if that suited you, of course.'

'Wow, that sounds great!' I replied, nodding keenly. At last *we* would have the chance to see some *motus* too...

'Sure does,' Mike agreed.

This mutually satisfactory scheme continued throughout our stay: Warren took us on occasional boat trips around the lagoon, and he borrowed Hilda to transport his guests from time to time. It was delightful to have the opportunity to explore the beautiful *motus* and beaches for day trips, and we enjoyed meeting his *papa'a* visitors too. It helped to expand our otherwise cramped world-view at the time. Our arrangement concluded very conveniently, with him buying Hilda from us when we left the island in late 1989.

Steve, another Kiwi, dropped over to our house shortly after our arrival and introduced himself to us. He invited us to his property where he had lived for decades with his local wife Poro, while most of his numerous adult offspring lived in New Zealand. Now in his 60's, he'd originally come to the island to do mechanical repairs on flying boats and planes in the 1950's, and they had set up a small farm on Poro's family land.

'Come out on Saturday if you'd like,' he said, 'I've got a nice crop of pineapples at the moment, so you're welcome to have a few.'

'That'd be wonderful,' I replied appreciatively. Fresh fruit in addition to bananas and pawpaws was an exciting prospect indeed, so we visited them on the following weekend, and from time to time after that. Steve and Poro always welcomed us warmly and were generous with their home-grown produce and practical assistance whenever we got in touch.

~

As well as the minimal shops on offer, we had also noticed the lack of places that provided meals or entertainment on Aitutaki, but we made the most of the few that were available whenever we could. Island Night was definitely the high spot of the week and was held every Friday at the Rapae, a restaurant and bar that also included some guest accommodation. Bonita assured us that we'd see and hear the best dancing and drumming on the island there, so we went with her for an evening out soon after our arrival.

As we entered the open-air restaurant with its thatched roof and simple decor, we bought a meal that had been cooked in a ground-oven, an *umukai*. The locals who were part of the evening's show were dressed in their traditional outfits and *eis*, and looked out at the audience with understated pride. At a signal from one of the leaders, eight or nine men began to drum complex rhythms on a variety of different-sized drums. Groups of women stood beside them chanting or singing lilting melodies, accompanied by guitars and *cocophones* (ukuleles made from halved coconut shells). The adults performed first, but it was also fascinating to see the youngsters getting into the action too. Young men, who had carefully honed their dancing skills from early childhood, performed their bold rhythmic stamping, while the girls swayed with iconic hip undulations.

We saw numerous Māori there as well and they encouraged us and the few other *papa'as* present to join in – probably just to laugh at our vastly inferior skills at traditional dancing! One of the locals explained that competitions occurred from time to time and the winners went on to Rarotonga, New Zealand and even Australia, to display their talents to wider audiences in the region. The whole evening was really good fun, made even better by knowing that the islanders would have done it all, whether *papa'as* were present or not – and it would have been just as loud, proud and brilliant.

~

It had been a difficult few months as we had tried to settle into island life. The kids had been sick with childhood bugs, so we were all sleep-deprived and grumpy. We'd found that, although our work was generally straightforward, there was the constant background uncertainty of a sudden knock on the kitchen door or the revving of an ambulance in our driveway to throw us into uncharted medical challenges.

After a particularly gruelling week, we decided to try Rino's – the only place where we could occasionally buy fish and chips. Back in Australia, we probably wouldn't have dressed up to go to a 'fast food' outlet – but since this was the only venue of its kind on the island, we rose to the occasion. Rhiannon insisted on selecting her own clothes and they proved to be a rather peculiar combination. Since we were all getting hungry though, we let her get on with it, since interfering with the choices of a three-year-old would have slowed her down intolerably.

'I wonder if they'll have real chips this time,' Mike said when we were all in the car at last.

'I sure hope so,' Rhiannon replied as we drove down the road, 'I don't like the other kinds as much.'

'True,' I agreed, 'But if breadfruit or sweet potato is all that they've got, I sure won't mind.'

'I guess the other consideration is whether they've been fishing lately,' Mike continued to muse, 'After all, you can't have fish and chips without the fish.'

Rhiannon considered this quietly. 'Mm, and my favourite sort is that bird kind – what's it called?'

'Parrotfish,' we replied in unison as we pulled up in front of the shop.

Looking through the car windows however, we noticed that all was in darkness and the shop doors were padlocked.

I groaned in dismay: 'Oh, no! I really needed some comfort food tonight. It's one of the few things that has kept me sane all day...'

Rhiannon started to cry and Thomas joined in, despite having little understanding of what was going on.

'What will we have for dinner now?' she wailed, 'I wore my

purple T-shirt and green shorts specially.'

Mike tried to turn back the tide of bitter despondency: 'Maybe I could make some toasties for us at home. Is there any cheese left in the freezer?'

'Mm, yes I think so – a little.' I tried to sound more enthusiastic than I felt at that especially low moment.

Then I had a sudden inspiration.

'Actually, I've got a good idea. Bonita told me that we can get *papa'a* food at the Akitua Resort, so we could go there tomorrow morning for a special breakfast, instead of tonight's fish and chips.'

My suggestion was met with a cautious reception by the rest of the family, as we travelled home for our meagre supper.

The Akitua Resort Hotel was the only place on the island that provided expensive accommodation and a quality restaurant – but its particular attraction for us was its all-you-can-eat English-style brunch for guests and local residents alike.

We arrived about eight o'clock the following morning, dutifully dressed up again and pleased to see food production underway. Our eagerness grew as we were directed to sit down at a classy table with serviettes and table decorations, while smartly dressed waitresses described the buffet options. But of course, the greatest attraction was the real *papa'a* food itself – it was just what we all needed, after the previous night's disappointments. We tucked in with enthusiasm to eggs and crispy bacon, and generous portions of fruit – it certainly helped to restore some semblance of equanimity for the busy week ahead.

After all, like so many others before us, we'd discovered that brewed coffee and sautéed mushrooms are truly effective remedies for a good many of the stresses and distresses of life.

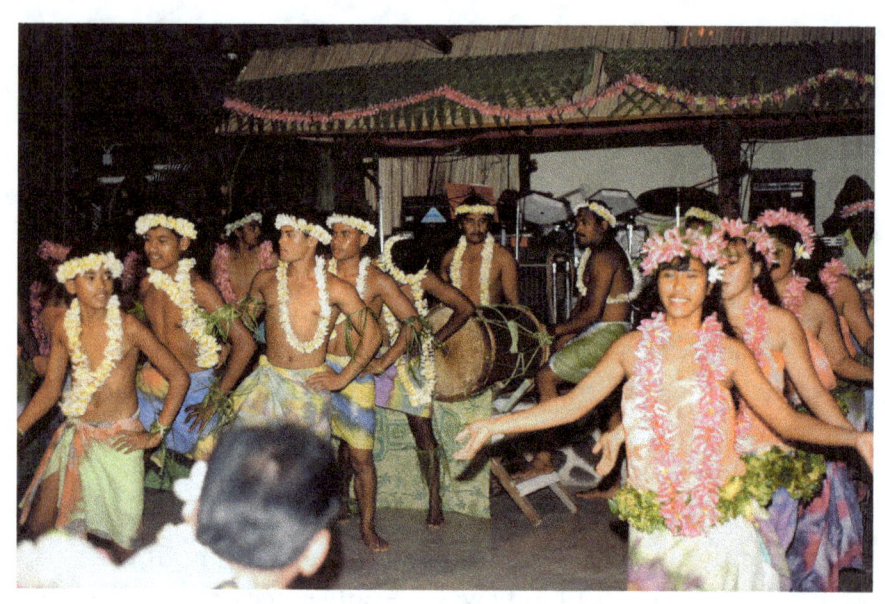

Island night at the Rapae Hotel

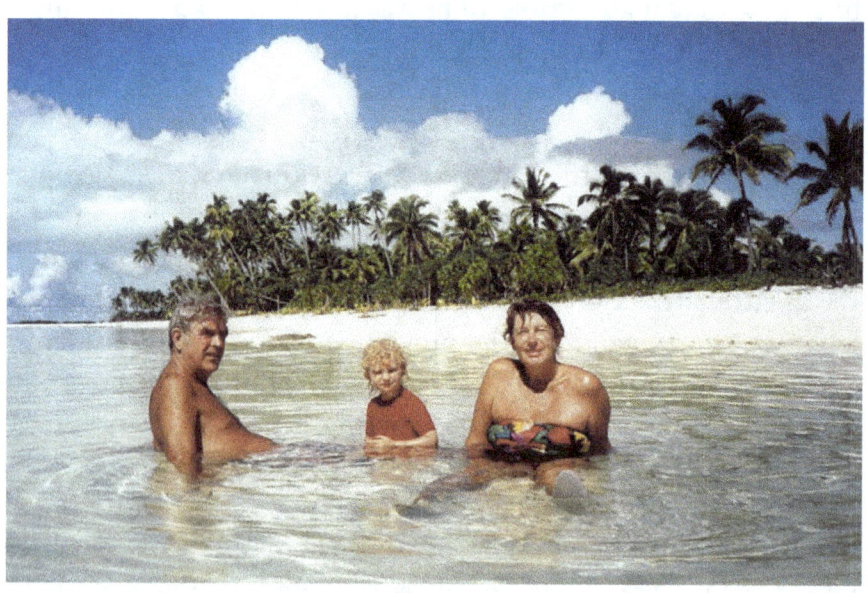

Motu trip with Mac, Rhiannon and Ena.

9 – Visitors (Part I)

One sultry afternoon in February, Mike held up a letter that had just arrived. 'I've heard from my parents and it's great news – they say they're coming to see us for three weeks.'

I looked up from my latest project. I had been able to borrow a sewing machine and was making some cushion covers to match our highly coloured (some might say, 'lurid') hibiscus-themed curtains. Thomas wasn't helping much as he crawled under the table, trying to remove the machine's foot pedal, while Rhiannon sat across the table from me, colouring in some bookmarks for her young *papa'a* friends next door.

'Great – when are they planning to arrive?' I asked, as I gently nudged Thomas aside.

'Mm – let's see,' he checked the pages again, 'Oh yes, the middle of March.'

'Ah, so maybe we could have an early party for Rhiannon's third birthday while they're here,' I said with a smile.

'What's that?' our daughter chimed in, always ready to hear her name mentioned.

'Grandma and Grandad are coming to visit us in a little while and we could have a pretend birthday for you, so they can join in too,' Mike replied, 'Won't that be fun?'

'Yes, *yes, yes* –' she said with a crescendo of excitement, 'And they'll be our first visitors here too!'

'They sure will – and you'll need to help us to get ready,' I said, moving onto the practical implications; 'Maybe we could borrow a spare bed and mattress from the hospital to put in Thomas' room so that you could sleep there, and then they could use the two single beds in your room.'

There were plenty of details to arrange as we looked forward to welcoming Mac and Ena, as well as showing them around 'our island.' I washed and sorted sheets and spare linen and we hired some local high school girls to clean our 338 louvres (yes, I counted them all). When we'd arrived on Aitutaki, the screens along the front of the house had been badly torn, allowing an occasional drunk passer-by to stick their arms between the louvres – quite a terrifying sight, especially at night. Thankfully, the hospital groundsmen had replaced the wire and that helped to keep out both inquisitive strangers and the numerous insect pests.

The evening before my in-laws arrived, Bonita and Father Luke called in, since it was our usual Tuesday meeting time. Rhiannon stuck her head through the doorway of her temporary bedroom and called out: 'Did I tell you that in a couple of whiles, Grandma and Grandad are coming?'

'Uh-huh,' Bonita replied with a grin, 'About fifteen times this week.'

'Oh,' said Rhiannon, 'Then let me show you how I've decorated their room.'

They duly admired the preparations and she was gratified enough to finally go to bed.

'I've brought some *tipani* too,' said Luke, putting a large box of Frangipanis on the table.

'Excellent,' I replied with considerable relief, 'We couldn't find many ourselves, and I've been too busy doing other stuff to look further afield.'

We were even more grateful when they both offered to sit at the dining-room table and thread the *eis* with us, while we sipped tea and shared our customary weekly debrief. The next morning, another huge box of *eis* appeared from the hospital staff, along with pawpaws and green coconuts called *nu*, so we ended up with an abundance of welcome gifts.

Greeting my in-laws at the airport was a joyfully teary occasion and they were thrilled with the many floral tributes that we placed around their necks. Mac and Ena had brought bags full of items that we had requested by earlier letters, as well as things they knew that we would appreciate: chocolate, hot cross buns, shock absorbers for the car, chocolate Easter eggs, toys and treats for the kids, more chocolate…

March was late in the wet season and we found it hard to tackle any serious work on the home front between 10 a.m. and 4 p.m. due to the clammy tropical heat, so the beach was definitely the best place to be. We called our favourite one 'Silcocks' Beach' after a family that had previously owned the small cottage adjacent to it. This beach was a lovely place due to its numerous coconut and pandanus palms, pristine white sand and shallow clear waters. The lagoon temperature was 27 degrees Celsius (80 degrees Fahrenheit) all year round, so it was invariably warm and inviting for kids and adults alike.

Rhiannon was keen to demonstrate to her grandparents how squeezing the fat black sea-slugs that lived on the sandy lagoon floor would make them squirt: the island equivalent of water pistols. The beaches had an abundance of shells and small crabs too, so building and decorating sand fortresses for the crabs provided another entertainment, as was relaxing in the shallows or snorkelling further out. We were often joined there by our *papa'a* neighbours – the volunteer family from next door and a Kiwi family from across the road – both of whom taught at the local high school and had two young daughters each.

On rare special occasions, various *papa'as* took us out in their motorboats to one of the *motus* for a day-trip. The *motus* were the fifteen tiny, mostly uninhabited islets within the lagoon that were generally used by the locals for fishing. The Akitua *motu* was the northernmost and closest to the Aitutaki mainland, and it housed the Akitua Resort Hotel that was accessed by a small barge. The only other *motu* that had a permanent dwelling on it was called Akaiami.

Each *motu* had its own particular features, with variations in size, shape and vegetation. The common attractions of *motu* trips for us included the spectacular beaches of fine white sand, having shade and shelter provided mostly by pandanus palms, so there was less risk of being hit by falling coconuts, as well as getting away from the incessant medical demands on the mainland. The snorkelling was brilliant in the nearby lagoon and, by trawling fishing lines behind the boat on the return trip, we were guaranteed a delicious range of fresh fish for dinner on our arrival home.

Our favourite *motu* was called: *Tapuaetai* (*Tai* = One, *Tapuae* = Foot, hence 'One Foot Island'), photos of which were used in Australia at that time to advertise the Cook Islands with the slogan: *'Visit heaven while you're still on earth.'* It was especially beautiful, with a wide sandbank connecting the two parts of the foot-shaped islet, and such vivid white sand that the surrounding lagoon water was a captivating blue-green colour.

There were various tales said to explain the background of

the name of One Foot Island, but the most popular one was this: *At some time in the distant mythical past, one Aitutakian tribe attacked another. A man and his young son escaped the battle by paddling their fishing-boat to an unnamed islet within the lagoon, where the father carried his son across the beach and hid him in a tall palm tree. The father then walked to the far side of the motu, swam back to his boat, and rowed to another part of the mainland to get supplies. When the attacking warriors searched the islet to look for escaped enemies, they found only one set of footprints traversing the motu. Assuming that no one had remained onshore, they left without discovering the boy. The father finally returned with provisions, and both father and son were safely reunited. So the islet came to be known as One Foot Island.*

The only *motu* that had a permanent private house on it at that time was Akaiami, and it was owned by one of the *papa'a* store-keepers, Dave and his Māori wife, presumably because it was part of her family land. There was no electricity, but it housed a kerosene stove, freezer and lamps. Water was provided by a rain-water tank and there was a simple long-drop toilet out the back. Mosquitoes on this *motu* were truly ferocious, so every bed was surrounded by nets. There were sleeping quarters for about twelve people and a large metal tub served for bathing purposes. The kitchen had a large wooden table with bench seats, and was well-stocked with pots, pans, and a motley assortment of old crockery and cutlery.

During my in-laws' stay, we had a three-day trip to Akaiami with Mac, Ena and Bonita. It was so good to get a few days of annual leave, and have beach trips, card games and barbecues on the shore with our freshly caught seafood. We also had a two-way radio to contact Dave to confirm the drop off and pick up arrangements.

During our time on Aitutaki, we had a total of four overnight trips to Akaiami for three to eight days each time – a much needed respite from the 24/7 demands that we so often dealt with on our doorstep at home. Day-trips that we made to other *motus* included ones to Moturakau, Maina, Papau and Rapota – all beautiful in their own unique ways.

Of course, our working life continued as the backdrop of our family's visit, and it proved to be as busy and challenging as ever. We often saw children who had been burnt by bumping their legs against the hot exhaust pipes of motorbikes when riding on the back, or gravel rashes from falling off. These injuries sometimes became infected and led to unsightly welts.

Fungal or bacterial skin infections were also extremely common through the long, wet summers. The latter, commonly known as 'school sores' or impetigo, were highly contagious and there was a major outbreak about this time. Sometimes, babies as young as six weeks of age were brought to Outpatients covered in these painful scabs that could lead to permanent scars if the condition was more chronic or severe. Early treatment with skin washing and antiseptic creams usually resolved the lesions quickly; but if delayed, oral and occasionally intravenous, antibiotics were needed to prevent further spread.

Mike continued to be busy with obstetric deliveries too, especially on nights and weekends. Of course, newborns can't read calendars or clocks, so they come whenever they are good and ready – regardless of other people's plans or need for sleep!

A few weeks after his parents' arrival, Mike was called to Outpatients one evening to see a local man who had been involved in a serious road accident. He had fallen heavily from his motorbike and had broken multiple ribs on the right side of his chest. An X-ray confirmed the fractures and showed that he had also accumulated a large amount of fluid in his right chest cavity. The fluid was compressing his lungs, making it difficult for him to breathe, and he was in significant pain.

After giving him a Morphine injection, Mike inserted a large-bore cannula and tubing known as a chest drain between the man's ribs and, after draining out 1.5 litres (3 pints) of blood and fluid, the islander's breathing improved considerably. With bed rest and analgesics, his rib fractures gradually repaired. The fellow was relieved when the drain was removed several weeks later and he could finally go home.

~

On the last weekend of my in-laws' visit, we were at home on a quiet Saturday morning. Ena was helping Rhiannon with a jigsaw puzzle, while Mac was building towers of wooden bricks with Thomas, when the phone rang.

'Uh-huh,' Mike said, 'Ok, no problem, I'll send the ambulance to the wharf to collect you at about 10 a.m.'

I looked up from the sewing machine where I was making T-shirts and shorts for the kids. 'What's the story?'

'A different kind of case this time,' Mike said, 'That was the ship's doctor from a cruise liner that was passing just north of us. Apparently, a woman passenger has had a fall and he thinks she's got a wrist fracture. He wondered if they could use our X-ray machine to check it out.'

'Mm – that *is* an unusual problem. We don't get too many high-class customers here, do we?' We exchanged a smile and I resumed my sewing.

Mike rang the hospital to arrange for the ambulance to collect the passenger, doctor and a ship's officer at the wharf, and he joined them at the hospital soon afterwards. The ship's medic Dr Frank, a delightful man with a softly-spoken American accent, was intrigued with the Korean War vintage American field army

X-ray machine that we had, and the fact that we still had to hand-develop our own films. While waiting for the X-rays to dry, Mike showed him around the hospital.

'Well, you really have to be on your toes here,' the doctor commented; 'There's no one else to pick up the pieces when things get messy, huh? And your working conditions are hardly world class.'

'Yes, you're right,' Mike replied. He related some of our recent challenging cases and Dr Frank gave a whistle of admiration.

'I definitely think your job's harder than mine. You take the idea of holistic care to a completely new level!'

The X-rays showed that the woman had fractured both of her adjacent right wrist bones, so Mike applied a plaster cast and sling. He found her some Paracetamol and helped her out to the waiting ambulance. Dr Frank gestured towards the X-ray machine and bandages, as he drew out some paperwork from a folder: 'So what do we owe you for all of this?'

'Well, all medical care in the Cook Islands is free,' Mike explained, 'So we can't really accept any payment.'

'Are you sure?'

This seemed to be unheard-of in the older man's experience and he was quite incredulous. Mike nodded and smiled, and the medic stepped outside to speak with the officer who had accompanied them. He returned shortly afterwards to the treatment area, where Mike was cleaning away bandages and a basin of water.

Dr Frank smiled: 'Hey there, we want to be able to thank you for all you've done. It's Saturday and you've had to come to work specially to help us out here. We thought maybe we could bring you and your family back to the ship for lunch so that we can show y'all some hospitality and appreciation for everything.'

Mike was very touched, but then frowned as he thought of

a small complication.

'Well that's very kind of you, but my parents are visiting us from Australia at the moment, and this is their last weekend here. We can't really leave them for the day.'

Dr Frank waved his hands expansively.

'No problem,' he said, 'They're welcome to join us too. How about we send the ship's tender back to the port at 12:30 p.m. and give y'all a ride to the ship?'

Well *that* was an offer too good to refuse, so Mike readily agreed. The ambulance ferried the ship's visitors back to the wharf and Mike came home with the exciting news.

At the appropriate time, the inflatable boat roared back to the wharf to collect us all, now properly attired for the occasion and thrilled at such an unexpected treat. We bounced through the reef passage and out to the enormous vessel, where we were welcomed aboard by the captain, various officers and Dr Frank. We had an impromptu tour of the ship's facilities, feeling overawed as we considered just how disparate our current humble islander lifestyle was, compared with the opulence of this floating resort.

Being led into the dining area was naturally the high point, especially for Rhiannon, who could scarcely contain herself with the thrill of so many culinary delights. The buffet was more extensive than any that we'd ever seen, with all kinds of multicultural foods on display.

Having always had an unusual palate for a two-year-old, she exclaimed with great excitement, 'I know what I'm going to have first – Greek salad!'

'Mm, well it certainly wouldn't be top of my list,' I murmured to Ena, 'Waldorf is much more to my liking – and coleslaw too – especially since I haven't even laid eyes on a carrot for months!'

We all roamed around the dining room, agonising over

the final decisions of what to eat. Too many meal options had hardly been a problem since our arrival on Aitutaki, and it was unlikely to become one anytime soon. The desserts were gloriously sumptuous and definitely worth going back for second helpings…

Thomas was now ten months old and had little interest in solids, preferring breastfeeds as his dietary staple. Dr Frank had grandchildren of his own and related warmly to our kids. Sitting at a table with Thomas on his lap, he tucked a serviette into his jumpsuit and proceeded to spoon small serves of ice-cream into our son.

'You're gonna like this, m' boy,' he said with a friendly grin.

At first, I was aghast that our son was being fed such contraband at his tender age. *(What would the Canberra Nursing Mothers' Association have to say about such appalling practices?)* But since our presence on the ship was such a surreal experience, and the whole day one of pleasurable serendipity, I relented and said nothing.

And I must say, Thomas devoured the ice-cream with great gusto, as he and Dr Frank shared a mutual sense of delight, playing games with every anticipated spoonful, cooing and chattering and exchanging smiles and gentle chuckles together.

10 – Kaikais

We appreciated being invited to a *kaikai* during my in-laws' visit, as it gave them a chance to experience this kind of Māori celebration for themselves. '*Kaikai*' means 'eat, eat' and that was definitely one of the main attractions of these events!

As it turned out, this particular feast was one of the biggest that we attended during our posting and, rather surprisingly, it commemorated the official opening of some new concrete tennis and basketball courts. Apparently, these had been planned for years following an extensive process of fund-raising. The construction had also taken quite some time, so the final outcome was considered worthy of a huge ceremony.

We discovered the general principle that the more significant the occasion, the more elaborate the feast and arrangements began weeks in advance of the celebration. *Kaikais* seemed to be one of the things that islanders took really seriously and, once the date was announced, they swung into action with considerable enthusiasm.

Firstly, a temporary structure was built adjacent to the new courts: it was roofed with woven pandanus palm leaves and supported by a bush-timber frame. Numerous trestle tables and bench seats were set up shortly before the event, and the poles and tables were decorated with copious quantities of hibiscus, *tipani* and *Tiare Maori*. Fruits were also set out on the tables in colourful displays: watermelon, bananas and pawpaws being the most popular, followed by oranges, custard apples and mangoes when these were in season.

Most cooking took place in ground ovens called *umus* or *umukais* in the tradition of countless generations of Polynesians, since naturally metal cooking pots had not been available in their ancient culture. For convenience, *umus* were usually excavated near the site of the planned ceremony. The earth floor was lined with rocks and shells, then wood and dried vegetation was added, and lit about twelve hours before the *kaikai*. Butchered meats (usually chicken, pork, goat and fish) and vegetables (taro, breadfruit *(kuru)*, sweet potato *(kumara)* and arrowroot) were wrapped in green banana leaves and laid on the hot rocks. A popular pudding called *pok'e*, made from arrowroot pulp and mashed bananas, was also wrapped in leaves and cooked with the rest.

Further broad sheets of banana leaves were then placed on top, followed by a final layer of vegetation. The whole arrangement was left to cook for many hours, and only dug up once the *kaikai* was about to start. Food prepared in this way was tender, juicy and truly delicious: it was certainly a great way to feed a crowd!

We arrived at the venue in the early afternoon, dressed in our best clothes and warmly welcomed by the village elders, who presented us with fragrant *eis*. As we were led to our seats, along with the other honoured guests, the kids wriggled with restless energy, keen to get on with things as soon as possible.

Fortunately, there was some chopped watermelon within easy reach on the tables, so we passed some slices to the kids to eat, as the large crowd of two-hundred or so islanders took their places. Those assisting ferried out massive portions of hot food from the nearby *umukais* and laid them along the centre of the tables, while most of the serving and eating was done by hand.

The ceremony began with a long and all-inclusive grace delivered by the invited clergy, and was followed by eating in the strict order of traditional Māori status: the first being the invited guests and honoured community members; second were the men; thirdly, the women; and finally, the local children. Since we were among the guests, we had no choice but to eat first.

'Come on Rhiannon, have some chicken and maybe some of this *kumara*,' I said softly as I scooped up a few portions by hand onto her mat-plate made from a small banana leaf.

'What's that grey stuff?' she said rather loudly, pointing to something in the centre of the table with a suspicious frown, 'It looks really yuk.'

Her words were clearly audible in the surrounding silence, making it impossible to hide this childish deficiency of social etiquette.

'I think it's a kind of taro,' I whispered with embarrassment, 'But you don't have to have it if you don't want to.'

Thomas had a negligible interest in solids at the best of times, and generally treated most food as an alternative form of play-doh, so he began to pound some pawpaw with his hands and smeared it into his hair. I blushed at these appalling table manners, so clearly displayed to the watching crowd. While trying to wipe him down with a handkerchief, I encouraged him to have some sips of green coconut juice called *nu*, to distract him from any further disgusting food-play.

Nu provided the usual drink at *kaikais*, as *papa'a* alcohol was not permitted. Although it was technically illegal, islanders often made their own pungent liquor by fermenting a wide range of fruits; and sometimes Māori carrying large buckets of homebrew could be seen wandering around the island in various stages of intoxication. But these beverages were for informal consumption only and were definitely taboo at *kaikais*.

Mike's parents Mac and Ena, though feeling quite self-conscious, tucked into the unfamiliar flavours with enthusiasm, especially enjoying some of the coconut cream side-dishes made from *okaru* – the orange semi-mature coconuts. These went really well with slow-cooked fish and *pok'e*, making the tastes and textures truly gourmet.

Mike tried to make small talk with the local big-wig who sat alongside him, but this chap seemed more interested in devouring large mouthfuls of goat as rapidly as possible, so the excruciating quietness was only broken by the sounds of chewing and guzzling.

Thankfully, once those officiating sensed that we had eaten our fill, a discreet signal permitted the men to begin eating. The crowd visibly relaxed and began talking – a welcome relief after being the centre of attention in the tortuous silence that we'd had to endure.

'Would you like us to pack some food to take home,' said one of the serving mamas with a smile. None of the women or children had been permitted to eat yet, and we realised that, if we took the generous quantities of food that were offered, there would be less for the others to eat.

'No thank you,' I said, 'You've already been so kind – we've had plenty already. Please, enjoy the food yourselves.'

The mama inclined her head graciously and another signal indicated that now the women were permitted to eat.

As both a mother and a doctor, I found it challenging that

the local children always ate last, which meant that their diet was largely composed of starchy *kumara*, taro or bananas. We had already begun to notice through our work that many kids had medical issues related to inadequate nutrition, such as anaemia and poor weight gain – so we hoped that by declining the 'take-away *kaikai*' that was always offered to guests, the local youngsters would get the benefit of more protein and iron-rich foods.

Kaikais were made up of a curious blend of Māori traditions and religious elements. Having begun with prayers, these ceremonies were invariably followed by numerous long speeches that were always given by men. The hard-court ceremony had about thirteen in all, with island leaders, sportsmen, builders, teachers, doctors and pastors all having their say. Mike soon learned a patter of Māori phrases that he moulded into a template of multi-occasion speeches. These were generally well received – partly because they were humorous, but also because they were mercifully short.

Our kids were getting well and truly over things by the second speech, so I took them for a walk around the outer rim of seated guests. We found a cluster of children playing together on the grass and chewing on *uto* – the crunchy hard coconut.

'Let's sit here for a while,' I said and the local kids made a space for us to join in. Rhiannon took off one of her *eis* and placed it around the neck of one of the little boys, who laughed with delight at her gesture of friendship. He passed her some *uto* and she gnawed it with the others.

'Wait here for a minute,' I said to our kids, and quietly walked back to our seat. On the table I found some chicken, meat and fish, and wrapped them in a spare leaf mat.

'Here – try some of this,' I said to the children on my return, and placed my finds on the banana leaf in the centre of their circle. The kids looked up with gaping eyes and exclamations of wonder.

'Go ahead – it's for you!' I smiled and nodded as they grabbed pieces of food off the mat without further delay, chewing with enthusiasm. The joy that this small gesture gave was humbling – and rather unexpectedly, Rhiannon joined in too. It seemed that everyone's appetites improved when eating together with friends. I went back and found some more food that was also hastily devoured by them all.

The verbose speeches finally came to an end and were succeeded by two coconuts being smashed with machetes by the officiating clergy – one at either end of the court – in a curious symbolic baptism, as the nuts split open and the clear juice spilled out. Long and prayerful entreaties were then offered by them both, asking for blessings, success and safety for all using the facilities. The *kaikai* culminated with the two priests, attired in their customary formal garb, playing an inaugural tennis match. It was an abbreviated affair, with a dearth of skill in evidence on either side of the net – but the gathered crowd keenly applauded.

The ceremony concluded with many locals, carrying all manner of bats and balls, streaming onto the courts and enjoying wildly spontaneous games themselves. The group of kids around us jumped up and joined in the fun as well, holding hands with ours and dancing with unconstrained excitement together. The facilities were thereby well and truly christened: a fitting conclusion to such a lavish and entertaining *kaikai!*

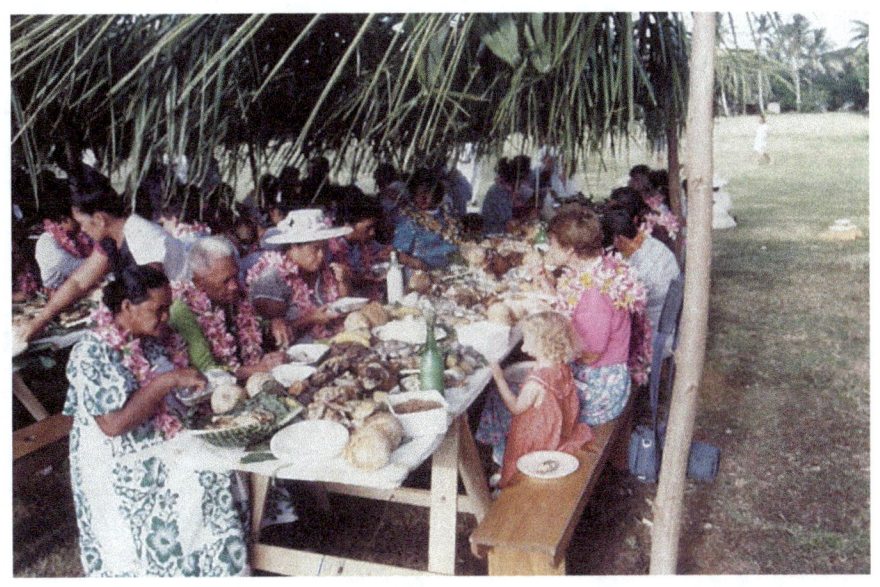

A *kaikai* with Rhiannon and Ena on front right-hand side.

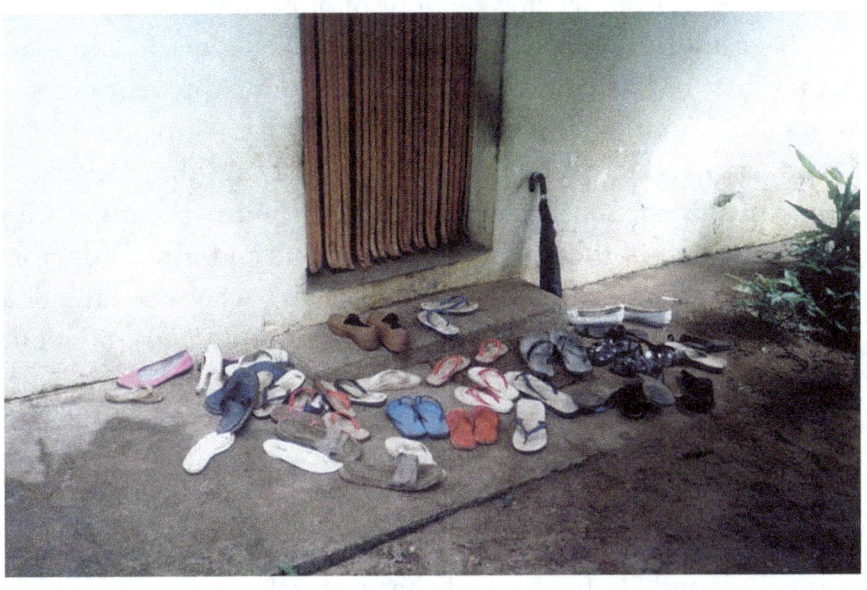

Our kitchen doorstep – so many visitors and/or patients as usual!

11 – The Tutaka

It was a clear cool morning in May, so refreshing after the long sultry wet season, when we set out in our car with the kids. We had been told to meet at the village hall at 8 a.m. on Monday, for the first of five days of home inspections. Apparently, three times each year an assessment of dwellings throughout the island was conducted, known as the Tutaka, and this one was to commence at the southernmost village of Tautu. The inspection team consisted of the Public Health officers and nurses, doctors (including our kids on the occasional days when we attended together) and a handful of others, making up a party of about ten people.

'Which part of Tautu do we check first?' Mike asked Moana, one of the Public Health officers, when we entered the village hall.

'Oh – the country areas,' he said with a distracted air as he handed around clipboards and charts of tick-boxes.

'Uh-huh,' Mike said and then whispered to me: 'Just before we move onto the city highlights.'

We smiled at each other and held hands with the kids while the most senior members of the team called everyone to order. One of the Public Health officers began the occasion, as most islander gatherings did, with prayers for safe-keeping and wisdom for the day ahead. Some speeches inevitably followed, but fortunately these were kept fairly short on this occasion. Mike then joined those on the ambulance while I followed in our car with the kids, who were now aged three and one. This meant that the three of us could make a discreet exit if the whole process proved to be overly tortuous.

As we drove to the outskirts of the village, we saw feral chickens and unfenced pigs roaming about, much to Thomas' delight, who enjoyed practising animal noises loudly from his car-seat. On reaching the first cluster of dwellings, we parked behind the ambulance and climbed out of the car to greet the villagers who warmly welcomed us. They shared some crunchy *uto* with us to snack on, and also *nu*, green coconut juice, that was delightfully refreshing to drink as the day warmed up.

The Tutaka gave us an opportunity to see the range of properties and living standards on the island. We were informed that Aitutaki had been severely affected by Cyclone Sally in January 1987 – in fact, the islanders told us that it was miraculous that no lives had been lost. Many houses had been destroyed or badly damaged, so some locals were still living in simple huts until their usual houses were repaired. These make-shift places, along with other permanent but similarly humble dwellings, were made of galvanised iron sheets for both walls and roofs, and had either dirt or sand floors. Long-drop toilets stood at the back of these properties and some had shared patches of cultivated root vegetables growing nearby.

It made me grateful that we lived in a house with multiple rooms, screened windows and a concrete floor.

'How do they do their cooking?' I whispered to Pua, the Public Health nurse. She led me around the back of a group of huts to a shared tepee, also made of iron sheets loosely abutting each other, with an open fire-pit centrally.

'The people from these houses cook together here and they use biscuit tins for their cooking pots. They can't afford saucepans and frying pans.' Pointing across to a single tap behind the cluster of dwellings, she added: 'That's used by all these families too – it's hard for them to stay clean and do their washing.'

My rusty washing machine was suddenly elevated to a place of reverence, as was our flush-toilet, stained bath and tiny fridge.

As we entered one especially humble hut, Mike and I gasped with amazement to see a group of people sitting on the bare floor, watching a video cassette of the American serial called 'Dallas' on their television. It would have been difficult to think of two more disparate extremes of materialism and social class on display in this dwelling, than those of the actors versus the viewers. Since Aitutaki had no TV transmission at this time, our kids had had no access to this entertainment for the past four months. They joined the locals on the sandy floor, intrigued by the programme. A marked sense of dissonance overwhelmed Mike and me, as we stared at the scene from the doorway.

Perhaps this medium fed the increasing trend of islanders to leave their villages and move to New Zealand to seek paid employment there. Some may have been tempted to pursue the possibility of improved financial rewards and social status by heading west. But for many, this dream remained elusive: it seemed that few actually found the prosperity they sought, whilst mourning the loss of their island communities and traditions, in this new country. Apparently, their automatic New Zealand citizenship had proved to be a mixed blessing for a large number of islanders.

For those who remained behind, there was a reduced population on their islands. During our posting, the entire Māori population in the Cooks was about 18,000, but this has apparently diminished in the decades since. One important benefit that locals had on their home islands was their inheritance of family land – an asset that was uniquely preserved for the owners, since no one could buy or sell their land. This gave Māori people the security of having a place to build a home and to supplement their food supply by growing crops, raising small livestock and fishing in the lagoon, regardless of whether or not they were formally employed. So, although local salaries were often low-grade, most islanders could sustain their families through this valuable resource. We had also noted that those who stayed on the island tried to protect their subsistence lifestyle and traditional cultural practices as much as possible – and Mike and I agreed that these were encouraging signs.

As we moved through the village to the more prosperous areas, we saw fenced enclosures for chickens, pigs, goats and occasionally cattle. The larger houses were similar to our own, being constructed of concrete bricks, with unscreened louvre windows and roofs of galvanised iron sheeting. These dwellings usually contained several large rooms, one of which generally held a long table with bench seats for mealtimes, and one or two others containing up to six double-beds in each room. This arrangement reinforced our observation that islanders did *everything* in the company of others. It was intriguing to imagine the variety of activities that could occur simultaneously in each of these rooms after dark...

Alongside this main building, there was often a separate hut that served as a kitchen, where cooking was done over an open fire with no chimney, using steel grills and occasionally western-style pans. Many dwellings had no electricity and relied on kerosene lamps at night. If they were fortunate enough to have running water, it came through a single tap into another small unroofed hut in the yard that served as both laundry and bathroom. Toilets were almost always long-drops at one end of the property, with fragments of banana leaves serving as convenient biodegradable toilet paper. There was also a space in most yards reserved for their *umukais*, and these were kept busy during the Tutaka.

I pulled up in front of a large house behind the ambulance, and the householders, who had evidently been sweeping their yard with stiff palm fronds, threw these aside and welcomed us warmly into their home. It was immaculately tidy, and colourful *tivaevaes* (hand-embroidered bedspreads) covered the numerous beds along with matching cushions that were also sewn in bright traditional floral patterns.

The householders led us into a dining area where yet another small *kaikai* awaited – with fish, chicken and root vegetables all steaming on a long trestle table. We sat down on the adjacent bench seats, and a protracted grace was uttered by the head of the family, followed by an invitation to eat our fill.

'It's not easy to tuck into more food at 11 a.m. when we've been to three *kaikais* already,' I murmured to Mike.

'Mm, I think pacing yourself is the key,' he whispered back as he took a small piece of chicken from the banana-leaf platter.

Rhiannon rolled her eyes at the sight of a further abundance of Māori food and looked around the room for something else to do.

'Why don't you go outside to the backyard and play with the kids there?' I suggested and she wandered off.

'And anyway, it's pretty hard to write anything negative on the assessment forms when they're feeding us so well,' Mike said softly with his mouth full.

'Yes,' I whispered in reply, 'Maybe that's the plan...'

Most of the Tutaka team were able to consume remarkable quantities of food, regardless of how many *kaikais* they'd already attended that morning, but we could only manage a few mouthfuls before heading out into the backyard.

I carried Thomas on my hip and complimented the family on their beautiful garden. Hearing some laughter from overhead, I looked up to see a few local boys of about six years of age at the top of several coconut palms. They drew out the machetes that had been thrust through the waists of their tiny shorts, and adroitly wielded them, lopping off green coconuts and clambering down to claim their prizes.

'They good at getting *nu* for the *kaikai*, huh?' their mamas bragged indulgently, as the youngsters sliced off the tops with further skilful swipes or stabbed the small holes in the nuts, the *mata*, so that the clear juice spilled out.

'Yes,' I replied with a tepid smile, stepping backwards to avoid the wide-swinging sharp blades, 'They're very clever indeed.'

My eyes alighted on a large bed of steaming coals in one corner of the garden where rubbish was being burned, since there were no garbage services on the island. Rhiannon and her new friends were running around it as they chased some feral chickens.

'Ah...' I tried not to shriek, but Mike quickly ran over and pulled our daughter aside.

'Hey, how about you play in – that corner?' he said, pointing to another part of the yard.

But then we spotted the large buckets and basins of water there – probably for washing or watering purposes. Some Māori toddlers crawled and cruised around these and Thomas wriggled hard, wanting to join in. I handed him to Mike, not prepared to lower him to the ground in front of these tempting, but possibly lethal, play-things.

I looked around again, trying to suggest somewhere else for Rhiannon to play, and observed the barbed-wire washing-line, conveniently hoisted to about 1.2 metres in height – just about right for an older child to collide with, and lacerate their vital neck arteries.

I felt myself fighting a sense of rising panic as I silently pondered: *How do these families survive? And how do I give them feedback about all of these potential dangers?*

Our roles in the Tutaka appeared to be limited to congratulating the Māori on their gardens, houses and *tivaevaes*, imbibing ridiculous quantities of food, and responding to the inevitable speech fests with our own halting contributions. If we noticed any problems, it seemed that we were expected to politely ignore them and move onto something we could commend instead. Being openly critical was definitely a cultural taboo, especially when we were being so liberally fed!

I urged Mike to lead the kids back through the house so that I could get them into the car and head for home.

As we passed through the main room of the house on our way out, I noticed a shelf near the front door that I hadn't seen when we had entered. In the middle, in pride of place, sat a large glass jar filled to the brim with pills and capsules of every imaginable kind and colour. Presumably, these had been handed out by hospital staff at some point in the past, but not actually ingested by the householders, who seemed immensely proud of their collection. But I shuddered at the thought that, as folk came and went, they could simply grab and swallow a random handful from the container, hoping that any unwanted symptoms they suffered would soon disappear. Of course, the concoction that they took could lead to yet another domestic hazard with life-threatening consequences...

We quickly got out to the car and I drove the kids home after the highs and lows of the morning. Later, as I sipped on a restorative cuppa, I considered the buoyancy of the Māori people as well as their wide-ranging priorities and living standards. It was humbling to witness their sense of pride in their possessions and traditions, and their resilience in the face of an almost endless array of ancient and modern perils.

Reflecting on all that I'd seen at the Tutaka that day, I silently shook my head and smiled to myself with a mixture of keen admiration and lively amusement.

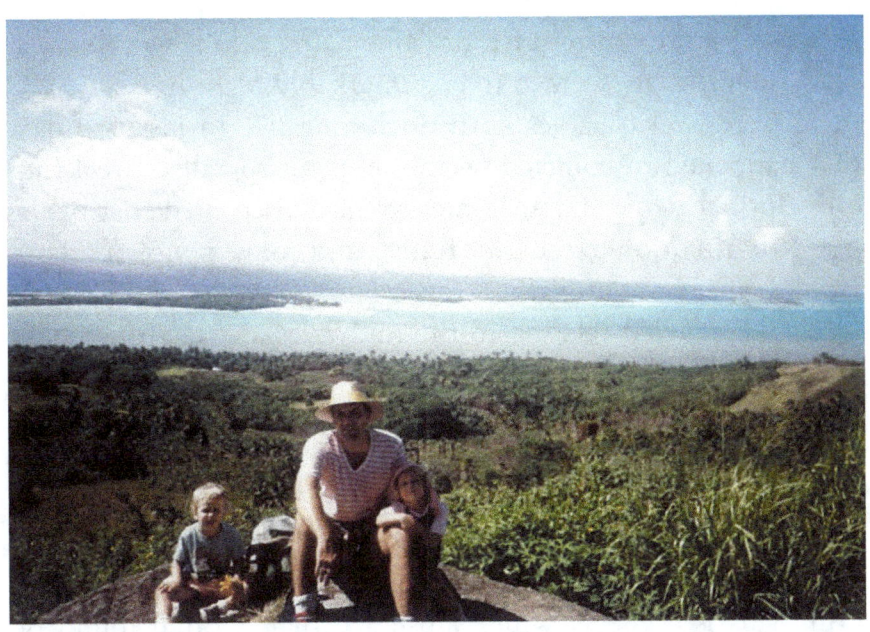

Mike with the kids on Maunga Pu, Aitutaki's highest hill - from which we could see the Pacific Ocean in every direction.

12 – Different Deliveries

Obstetrics took up much of Mike's after hours' workload, as the birth rate seemed to be remarkably high. In May, 1988 there were twelve babies born, including five in just two days that happened to coincide with one of his so-called 'weekends off'. Both at work and at home, we had discovered that babies pay little attention to the time frames and convenience of others, either before or after birth!

Mike enjoyed relating to the midwives and chatting about various features of normal versus worrying deliveries. He was keen to see how they handled the island's obstetric demands, having in mind the OSB caution about not de-skilling local practitioners by his interventions. After watching Abi, one of the midwives, deliver a healthy *pepe* (baby) early in our posting, Mike drew her attention to the coating of vernix on the infant's skin. This is a cheesy white substance that is often found on babies when they are born close to their due date: it's a natural agent that protects the foetal skin from being damaged by continuous exposure to amniotic fluid in the womb.

'Hey Abi – look at this beautiful vernix,' he exclaimed, pointing to the newborn's arm that was copiously smeared with it; 'The people who make cosmetics wish they knew how to make this stuff – and midwives back home love to rub it onto their hands.'

Abi nodded thoughtfully and then said: 'But it's better for the *pepe* when it's green, isn't it?'

Mike's smile sagged into a frown. When unborn babies are experiencing serious oxygen deficiency or other trauma in utero, they empty their bowels of meconium: a greenish black substance that appears with the amniotic fluid during delivery. Meconium-stained liquor is therefore a worrying sign of high-level foetal distress during the birth process. Mike suddenly realised that this experienced midwife was not aware of the significance of 'the green stuff' and her comment that its presence was 'better for the *pepe*' concerned him deeply.

While carefully explaining to Abi what meconium indicated, he went on to say: 'In future, I want to be called in for *all* the deliveries, even the ones that you midwives are doing – just so I can check on the babies afterwards, ok?'

Abi shrugged complacently and, with a brief nod, went on wiping down the newborn and handing her to her mother.

~

We had just arrived home from a late afternoon beach walk with the kids when the ambulance drove into our driveway, as it did so often.

'Mama in labour ward,' the driver said with a grin, waving to me and the kids as we pulled off our beach-shoes. I nodded back with a weary smile – I was going to have to do the bathtime-dinnertime-bedtime routine on my own again, it seemed. I also noticed the kids dragging sandy wet towels across the doorstep into the kitchen and frowned – another mess to clean up, as well.

Mike shrugged grimly at me and climbed into the ute, as the ambulance blared out a song from the local radio station. The bouncy rhythms and predictable chord sequences of the island melodies all sounded remarkably alike, he thought – but of course it was impolite to point this out to those who hummed along to the tunes, including the driver who cheerfully tapped in time to the beat on the steering wheel. Mike sighed as the vehicle hauled its way up the hospital hill.

As he entered, he recognised one of my friends called Tuka on the labour ward bed. She was a Māori young woman who had spent some of her adolescence in New Zealand. She was already sweaty, pale and groaning in considerable pain. The midwives alternately shouted and laughed at her, neither of which seemed to offer any great comfort to the distressed mama.

Mike took her by the hand and gave it a gentle squeeze. 'Hey Tuka, this is your first *pepe*, huh?'

She nodded as the tearing contraction slowly subsided.

'Not going too well, I see,' he added and she shook her head as tears tumbled down her cheeks.

'No, it's not. The pains started a few hours ago, but they're already feeling really bad.'

'It's ok, I'll put in a spinal block – that should help quite a lot.'

Tuka nodded before another powerful contraction had her focused on her breathing once again. The midwife Tua and matron Kata seemed ready to stay for the evening, as they brewed themselves tea and pulled up a chair on either side of the labouring mama. Often it was unclear as to whether their decisions to stay were professionally motivated, or simply an excuse for a long and gregarious chat. But either way, Mike was glad of their company, as he sensed he could be in for a long and difficult night.

Having gathered up what he needed for a spinal block from the dispensary, he put them into a kidney dish and returned to labour ward.

'Hey Mr Dr Browne, do you want a sandwich and some tea?' Tua asked, and he nodded keenly in response.

'Yes, that'd be great, thanks,' he said with a grin, 'I haven't had dinner so far tonight.'

She heaved herself upwards. 'Corned beef or baked beans?'

Mike cringed at the thought of cold baked beans – even in labour ward he had his standards. 'I'll have the tinned corned beef thanks.' She flicked her eyebrows as she disappeared from the room.

'Can you help me to position Tuka for the block?' he asked Kata. Together they sat her up and Mike inserted the syringe containing Heavy Nupicaine between her lumbar vertebrae: it combined a local anaesthetic agent with a dense glucose solution to make it sink to the lowest part of the spinal canal to numb the 'saddle region' of the mama's body. They laid her down after ten minutes and Tuka began to relax as her pain slowly receded.

Tua returned with a thick pile of sandwiches and a mug of tea.

Mike took a hungry bite and thanked her with his mouth full. The nurses laughed before resuming their conversation. When he'd finished eating, he checked on his patient again.

'How are you going, Tuka? You should be feeling a bit better by now, I think?'

She let out a slow sigh. 'Mm, yes I am thanks. It was really bad for a while there.'

Mike smiled. 'Yeah, they don't call it "labour" for nothing, do they?'

She nodded in agreement and gradually dozed off. He decided to do a few low-key tasks to fill in the evening as the nurses' prattle rose and fell, punctuated by noisy guffaws from time to time.

Every hour or so, he returned to check on Tuka's vitals and listen for the baby's heart sounds with a wooden ear-piece. The infant's heart rate dropped precariously from time to time, and he worried that this could indicate low-grade foetal distress. Sometimes he thought that his obstetric training was just enough to recognise when all was not going well, but not enough to solve each dilemma on the spot and with no back-up options available.

At times like this, labour ward felt like a very lonely and daunting place to be.

He tried to get occasional snatches of sleep between check-ups as the night wore on, but gnawing anxiety made it hard for him to relax. Eventually, in the early hours of the morning, he did an internal check and found that Tuka was fully dilated. However, despite the fierce exhortations of the midwives for her to push hard, amplified by a few sharp slaps, the weary mama's bearing down failed to expel her baby.

Mike knew by now that he would need to intervene to resolve the impasse. He had previously found a set of Neville-Barnes obstetric forceps lying around in a cupboard in the sluice room and it seemed that the time had come to use them. These implements were about the length of tyre levers or large barbecue tongs, comprising two large curved metal blades that clicked together. They operated like heavy-duty salad servers to secure either side of the infant's head and allow controlled traction to ease the baby out.

By now, the spinal block was wearing off – it should have

improved Tuka's ability to push, but only seemed to have made her pain worse, and she was rapidly becoming exhausted. After a few more minutes of failure to progress, he announced to the nurses, 'Ok, enough's enough. We're going to need the obstetric forceps. Can you get them ready please?'

Their garrulous conversation halted and with quick nods, they rose and went in search of the implements.

Mike spoke quietly to the weary mama: 'Tuka, I'm worried that your *pepe's* getting distressed because the labour's taking too long, so I'm going to use forceps to speed things up.'

She nodded forlornly, no doubt longing for the ordeal to end. He scrubbed and gloved up for the procedure, and mentally rehearsed the process of putting the forceps together and applying them to the baby's head.

After some delay, the midwives returned and, with great ceremony, handed Mike a surprisingly petite package. Looking puzzled, he tore open the wrappings to find a set of Bonney's dissecting forceps that were about the same size as a small pair of household scissors. In a moment of dismayed revelation, he realised that these most experienced of midwives on the island had never assisted with a forceps delivery. In fact, it seemed that they'd never even witnessed one either, nor even knew what obstetric forceps looked like.

This was far from ideal timing to make such a significant discovery. As usual however, he had no choice but to proceed regardless, and went with them to find the correct implements. While the midwives quickly cleaned them up, Mike mused on theoretical methods of trying to deliver a baby with a pair of dissecting forceps – it provided some brief entertainment to divert his attention away from the burden of anxiety that had dominated much of the night.

The midwives eventually returned with the clean equipment

and handed it to Mike. As he inserted some local anaesthetic and did a generous episiotomy, the nurses dropped their chins onto their chests and muttered passionate prayers for a successful outcome.

As they concluded, he carefully applied the forceps to the baby's head. Firmly heaving with the next few contractions, he finally pulled a healthy baby girl out into the world to the great joy of Tuka and everyone else present. Chatter and laughter filled the ward as the crying infant was passed around for all to admire, and Mike sat down to enjoy a few moments of gratitude and relief.

However, the elation of success was soon succeeded by the painstaking tedium of repairing the large episiotomy with our oversized suture materials. Fatigue sapped his concentration and he felt damp with blood-stains and sweat. It was finally done though, and he trekked back home as the new day dawned, to try to catch a few hours of sleep before another morning of work commenced.

In the early afternoon after Outpatients was finished, he checked on Tuka and her baby, along with the other in-patients. Asking how she was going, Tuka and the staff replied with typical Māori understatement that all was fine, although he noticed that the new mama looked rather pale. He's still not quite sure why he did so, but he pulled back the bed sheets and found the mattress and Tuka's lower body drenched in bright blood. She had clearly had a serious post-partum haemorrhage in the past few hours and needed an urgent blood transfusion.

Mike quickly called for the drivers and hospital technician, but was informed that the ambulance that had sounded far from robust on the trip up the hill the previous evening, was now no longer working at all and had been towed away for repairs. The other diesel-powered one was also unavailable.

He ground his teeth in exasperation: *Of course the ambulance would be broken down just when it was urgently needed...*

He arranged to have our car collected, and a driver used it to round up the technician who completed the basic cross-matching. After announcing appropriate donors, the driver was dispatched to collect them for donor-to-recipient transfusions over the next few hours. By nightfall, Tuka was looking much brighter and her bleeding had slowed to a trickle. She even managed to share some laughs with the nurses – a good sign under the circumstances.

Despite his mind-numbing weariness, Mike had a joke that he made to many of the mamas as he farewelled them following their deliveries, and he repeated this several days later to my friend:

'I'll see you here again next year.'

And sure enough, Tuka was one of the four women whom he successfully delivered twice during our islander posting.

~

Another birth ended up being memorable for all the wrong reasons, but he learned some important lessons along the way.

A teenage primip (first time mother) laboured long and hard through another protracted delivery, and Mike fretted over the slow progress that she was making. With the aid of a large episiotomy however, she finally gave birth to a skinny baby boy, whose breathing was patchy and shallow. His pale limp body heaved erratically and Mike quickly intubated him and air-bagged with oxygen until his breathing became more stable.

While concentrating on the resuscitation however, Mike gradually became aware at the edge of his consciousness of a sound that resembled a dripping tap. He turned around and saw blood tumbling from the mother's perineum into an expanding pool on the labour ward floor. The two midwives simply stood there, staring at the haemorrhage in speechless fear.

'Quick, take over with the baby!' Mike shouted to attract their attention and passed the air bag to one of the nurses.

He then shoved his right gloved hand into the mother's vagina while rapidly massaging her abdomen with his left, to try to induce uterine contractions.

'Can you *please* get some Syntocinon from the dispensary straight away?' he asked urgently.

The other nurse rushed out, and returned a few minutes later with the precious ampoule. He quickly injected the agent into the mother's thigh and, much to his relief, her bleeding gradually slowed.

Syntocinon is a synthetic form of the hormone Oxytocin and is used following a delivery to limit bleeding by stimulating contractions of the uterus. At this time on Aitutaki, Syntocinon was rarely given post-partum, even though this would have been a routine practice in most western hospitals by then.

Once the mama's bleeding had subsided, he checked for any other potential sources of the haemorrhage. Finding a large tear high in the vaginal wall that had presumably occurred during the difficult delivery, he proceeded to suture the ragged edges together.

By that time, the infant was breathing well, so Mike removed the endotracheal tube. He was also concerned that the baby boy may have aspirated contaminated fluid during the protracted delivery, so his last task for the night was to inject intramuscular Penicillin into the infant's tiny buttock.

Returning the following morning, however, he was distressed to see that the baby's injection site had transformed into an enormous bruise, equivalent in size to a third buttock. The baby looked pale and his heart-rate was very rapid – it seemed that he had lost a considerable amount of blood into the swollen area. Mike surmised that he had developed haemorrhagic disease of the newborn: a tendency to bleed due to Vitamin K deficiency after birth. Thankfully, Mike found some Vitamin K vials in the dispensary and inserted one of these into the *pepe's* thigh. The huge buttock bruise gradually settled over the following week or so.

Once the baby and mother had recovered from their various complications, they were discharged from hospital ten days later. From that time on, Syntocinon injections for mamas and Vitamin K for *pepes* became routine in labour ward – at least as often as Mike was present and the supply system allowed.

~

Assisting sick newborns was an ongoing challenge and Mike had to try some unorthodox techniques on several occasions.

Following a further difficult forceps delivery, he had to resuscitate a baby who was six weeks premature and weighed just four pounds (or 1.9 kg). The infant looked floppy and bluish, so Mike proceeded to intubate him with his smallest paediatric endotracheal tube. However, there were no appropriate-sized connecting parts to attach this tube to the large oxygen cylinders at the hospital.

Yet again, creativity was required.

Taking mouthfuls of oxygen from the cylinder himself, Mike gently blew them into the endotracheal tube, while carefully pinching off the baby's nose to ensure the oxygen went directly into his tiny lungs. He had to continue this for five minutes or so until the *pepe* became more pink and responsive.

Of course, the hospital had no humidicribs either, but the

little chap enjoyed snuggling up to a hot water bottle wrapped in a fluffy sheet that helped his body temperature to stabilise nicely.

The infant was too small to attach to his mother's breast for the first few days of life, so he had to have coconut *nu* juice or expressed breast milk through an eye dropper. After several days, he was able to start normal breastfeeding and rapidly put on weight, so that by the time he and his mother were discharged from hospital a month later, he was almost six pounds or 2.7kg.

We felt immensely gratified when things worked out better than we had expected – it helped to compensate for the various occasions when that certainly didn't happen. Those joyful sensations of success were always warmly savoured and caused our struggles to melt into mists of sweet oblivion.

~

Another evening, yet another occasion when the Toyota ambulance revved insistently in our driveway...

'Mama having *pepe* in Vaipeka,' the driver reported as he conveyed Mike to a collection of small dwellings on the edge of the village. The simple houses were close to one another and there was a cheerful atmosphere among the locals.

There they found the multiparous mother whose labour had developed so quickly that she was far too advanced to be transferred to hospital. Rather surprisingly, she was labouring on a large blue banana-ripening bag on the bare earth of her front porch. The village men and children kept their distance, but the neighbourhood women laughed and conversed with one another alongside the mother.

One of the women handed Mike a kerosene Tilley lamp, since these houses had no electricity. He assessed the mama's progress as accurately as possible under these spare conditions and found that she was close to full dilatation.

Between contractions, she chatted with those milling about, and it wasn't long before she was bearing down. By the shadowy lamplight and crouching on his haunches, Mike's gloved hands soon delivered a chubby baby girl. The assembly of villagers applauded and burst into spontaneous hymns to thank the Almighty for this healthy new life.

While waiting for the placenta to appear, Mike became aware of a strange bumping sensation against the back of his knees. After fumbling with the lamp and feeling with his hands, he discovered a baby goat nudging him and bleating softly – an unusual intruder even in this rustic home-birth situation! The locals laughed at Mike's surprise, yet somehow the kid fitted so well into the somewhat surreal events of the evening, that he joined in cheerfully as well.

The delivery was capped off by the driver offering Mike the padded passenger seat inside the warm cabin of the ambulance, whilst directing the mama and her newborn to the hard bench-seats on the back of the ute, to transport them to the hospital for post-natal care. The driver was indignant when Mike insisted on a swap and took the outside seat for himself.

He smiled about the whole episode, as the ambulance bumped along the winding unsealed road. As he looked up at the glowing silvery moon and felt the cool evening breeze on his face, he mused on the many small and whimsical wonders of this tiny island, tucked away in our modest fragment of a very large globe.

13 – Achievements and Amusements

Thomas began walking at ten months of age and within days was running everywhere. Since our house was situated on an open block adjacent to a busy street, we soon saw the need to corral him in, especially after finding him across the unsealed road on several occasions. Consequently, Mike promptly set to work constructing a hefty DIY fence in front of our house as our son's first birthday present, to preserve his young life for future birthdays.

Mike had packed various tools in the car before its departure from Canberra, and was able to borrow others from the hospital groundsmen or *papa'a* friends. He also sourced wood from cheap pallets at the local stores, as well as chopping down saplings from the bush behind our house. Sawing, hammering and attaching wire kept him busy whenever he was not at work, until he had made a fence across the front and sides of our yard. He even extended his talents to making hinged gates, as his skills and enthusiasm grew.

'It looks good,' I said as I admired the finished project and shook the posts to check how stable they were; 'What's next?'

He looked around cautiously to ensure that no little ears were listening in. 'Well, I've decided to make a wooden stove for Rhiannon's birthday in April.'

I smiled in response. 'Sounds great, she'd love that.'

'Yes, I hope so. I've found a few lids from Milo tins to use for the hot plates, and a handle from an old drawer for the oven door.'

Rhiannon was delighted with her gift on the morning of her third birthday and proceeded to cook play-doh cupcakes and mini-pizzas in the oven. Mike moved on to constructing more kids' furniture as well: a small low table with adjacent bench seats that our kids used daily for meals and playtime, especially when other youngsters came to visit.

Rhiannon was keen to join in with her own creations as well. She looked up from a sketch that she had done at her small table one morning. 'I want to make something, too.'

'Uh-huh,' Mike replied, 'What did you have in mind?'

She held up her diagram, but it was difficult to appreciate the finer points.

'Here,' she said firmly.

'Can you talk us through it?' I said, hoping to get a better idea of her plans.

She snorted indignantly and declared: 'Can't you see? It's a cockroach spreader – for hitting them with.'

Mike smiled warmly. 'Actually, that would be very helpful indeed.'

So with our assistance, she completed her device and put it to frequent use against the endless assaults of these household pests. Having been forewarned about the formidable population of cockroaches in the house by the Vandermoezels, we had brought a wide range of surface sprays and baits with us in our car and placed them conscientiously around the house. But their numbers grew inexorably throughout our stay. In fact, we soon discovered that, far from being subdued by these poisons, the resilient creatures appeared to congregate and propagate right next to them.

Mike's constructions also included a wooden sewing table that doubled as an ironing board. When I was able to borrow a sewing machine, I had bursts of satisfying productivity since clothing was in short supply in the few island shops. I sewed T-shirts, shorts and track suits as the kids grew from one size to another, as well as smocked or stretch knit dresses for Rhiannon.

I learned further sewing skills when joining a nearby *Tivaevae* group, at the invitation of Tuka, one of my local friends. Sitting on the floor of a local village hall, the islander women showed me how to make the beautiful appliqué cushions and bedspreads that adorned their homes.

'This is the hibiscus pattern,' a mama said, helping me to cut it out for a pillow-case.

'They're very bright, aren't they?' I commented. The bold primary colours of the cloth seemed to ricochet around the room.

'Yes, we like the happy colours.' The mama smiled and the others murmured their assent appreciatively. I had already noticed that pastels didn't seem to suit the islander psyche in any context!

Sometimes Rhiannon came to the group as well with her own small projects, as did some of our *papa'a* neighbours. It was a good opportunity to develop a sense of camaraderie with the local women and to learn more Māori words and ways as well.

~

One afternoon, I was out in the car with our kids when we came across a group of villagers who were processing arrowroot on the back of a large truck. It looked interesting, so I pulled over and parked. Asking if we could watch, the good-natured locals made us welcome as they dug out the deep-rooted plants and cut off the leaves with machetes. They washed and chopped the thick roots into smaller pieces, then smashed the coarse fragments with wooden blocks or hammers. Then they strained the pulp through netting and separated the inner glutinous paste into large bowls from the fibrous outer layers.

The mamas tossed the husks onto the back section of the truck, where the village kids were playing. The youngsters invited Rhiannon to join in and of course she was keen, so I lifted her up and they moulded, pounded and tossed the husks to each other, inventing games and giggling in delight. I held Thomas on my hip and chatted with the locals.

Some of the mamas peeled and mashed bananas too and mixed them into the tubs with the arrowroot paste. Shovelling up large handfuls of the mixture, they carefully wrapped these mounds into parcels using green banana leaves, to cook in their *umus* for a forthcoming *kaikai*, producing the delicious dessert called *pok'e*.

I was fascinated with the islanders – whether fishing, cooking, dancing, drumming or creating, their many skills were impressive. Coupled with their insatiable capacity for enjoying themselves, I felt that we had much to learn from them.

~

Between Mike's work and mine, we gradually became aware

of the lack of good contraceptive advice on the island. Most girls became pregnant in their mid-teens, when young males 'found' the girls in secluded parts of the island or in their homes when their parents were out, and took full advantage of the circumstances. Whether these encounters were viewed as 'rape' by the locals was unclear – perhaps they saw it more as: 'Boys will be boys, and girls will be mamas,' and accepted it as fate.

Either way, we felt challenged to take a more active role in addressing the high rates of both youth pregnancy and sexually transmitted diseases. We found an unlikely ally in the form of Father Luke. Knowing the Catholic Church's opposition to contraceptive use, we hadn't expected our friend's support of our plans. However, he had witnessed numerous problems related to promiscuity among his parishioners and therefore encouraged our efforts to make this information more available.

Bonita also helped us to liaise with the executive staff at the High School, to organise some time-slots for sex education with the students. Our strategy involved separating the kids by gender, with Mike teaching the boys and me the girls. Mike used his sessions to explain the biology of reproduction and encouraged the boys to use condoms and have a considerate attitude towards females. I talked with the girls about reproduction and pregnancy, along with the ways that different contraceptives worked.

As with teenagers anywhere, both groups regarded the whole topic with a mixture of amusement, embarrassment and scepticism, but gradually curiosity got the better of them and they listened with interest. I particularly urged the girls to be proactive about self-protection, by staying close to friends when they were in lonely places around the island, carrying condoms and doing what they could to insist on more respect from males. I advised them that they could get individual contraceptive advice at the women's clinic if they wished, and assured them that they *could* have more control over their own fertility.

Empowerment seemed to be a novel concept for many of the girls – after all, most of them had seen their peers becoming pregnant early in life, regardless of their personal wishes or plans. I hoped that these sessions gave them a greater sense of self-worth, and encouraged them to make good decisions for themselves, and not view teenage pregnancy as inevitable.

Although it wasn't possible to assess objectively whether our input was 'successful,' we hoped that it would prove to be helpful, at least to some of the students.

~

While finishing up at the women's clinic one day, Pua was keen to tell me that she had been invited to attend an all-expenses-paid World Health Organisation (WHO) symposium on contraception that was being held in Fiji in the near future. Her comments reminded me that I had previously shown her my concise handbook on contraception.

'You know Pua, that book I showed you is in our office so that any of us can look up the latest contraceptive recommendations,' I said to her.

She nodded dismissively. 'Yeah, yeah, I know. But I can learn lots at a conference too.'

'Yes, I'm sure you can,' I replied, not wanting to dampen her sense of excitement.

'And the information they give is very up-to-date too,' she added carefully.

'Yes, of course,' I agreed, then thought of another idea: 'Would you like to run some education sessions with the nurses when you get back? By then, you'll have learnt some useful things at the conference to share.'

'Sure, sure,' she said hastily as she headed towards the door.

'Have a good time, and let me know how you go,' I called out as she disappeared from view.

Shortly after Pua's return, I saw her at work and asked about her experiences.

'It was really good,' she replied warmly, 'There were people from all over the Pacific and we had *kaikais* every night with food from every country group that was there.'

'Wow – it sounds amazing,' I said; 'How many people went?'

'I think about two-hundred altogether,' she said and added with pride: 'I was lucky to be asked to go, you know.'

'You sure were.'

It certainly sounded like an expensive and complex event for the WHO to have organised.

'Would you like to tell the other staff about what you learned?' I asked, 'I could present some information from my textbook too, if you wanted my help.'

'Ah, maybe – if I'm not too busy.' She sounded evasive and I was already learning that sharing information was not necessarily seen as a positive by everyone at the hospital.

She gathered up the infant scales for the baby health clinic and was heading out when I remembered to ask her: 'By the way Pua, what's one thing you learnt about contraception while you were at the conference that you didn't know before?'

She seemed momentarily flustered by my question and jiggled the scales impatiently before breaking into a grin: 'That's right – they're going to make a pill for men one day, so that the women don't have to take them.'

'Ah – I see.'

I smiled to myself as she bustled out. Even then, and still thirty years later, the 'male contraceptive pill' is only a theoretical construct. It was hardly a useful piece of knowledge to have picked up from the event or to pass on to the other staff. As I shook my head, I recalled that my simple but informative handbook sold for a mere fifteen Aussie dollars – a far cry from the lavish international conference.

We often wondered what interventions were most likely to be effective in improving health outcomes in developing nations. Teaching local health workers current recommendations in their own context was the most likely to be useful for them and their communities, we thought, especially when it was done by those with practical experience and simple readily available resources, rather than occasional high-cost events. However, at the end of the day that was only our opinion.

And after all – who knows?

~

One of our earliest projects after settling into our island home had been to have a thriving vegetable patch. Mike had been a keen gardener since we had first owned our own place in Canberra and he'd successfully supplied us with many home-grown veggies in the past. We had brought over packets of seeds and gardening implements to Aitutaki in our car, having heard from the Vandermoezels that these could prove useful. Despite our best efforts, however, most plants were either infected with horticultural diseases or rapidly devoured by bugs, birds, rats or roaming chickens.

Even when Thomas waved his arms hysterically and screamed: 'Bog off chooks!' there seemed to be little impact.

Apparently, we were doomed to lose most of our produce to heat, ferals or fungi, with only an occasional snow pea or lettuce leaf spared for our consumption. It was all quite disheartening.

We decided to wreak our revenge, at least on the fowls, by

setting up a chicken trap. This was composed of a one metre square wooden frame with wire on the top, elevated on one side with a stick to which ten metres of eight-pound fishing line was attached with a sturdy knot. Scraps of food were placed underneath and the fishing line was strung along the grass beyond the corner of the house, where we quietly awaited our prey.

Once an unsuspecting fowl had been trapped by a decisive pull on the line, it was beheaded, plucked and disembowelled. Most of the feral chooks were wiry little beasts – not at all like the hormone-stuffed sedentary ones that we had previously enjoyed back home – so we needed to cook them in our own back-garden *umu* for at least six hours. Then they were ready for electric oven-baking for another few hours, preferably with real potatoes if these treasures were available, and served with gravy. Even after all this, we'd be flossing our teeth for another few hours, to remove the sinewy remnants from around our gums.

So in total, a roast dinner could take up to ten hours from start to finish – certainly not to be undertaken lightly or by the faint-hearted.

~

When leaving Australia, we had packed a cheap hair-cutting set with our luggage, rightly anticipating that there wouldn't be regular hairdressing services available on Aitutaki. I had postponed learning how to use the electric shaver until our arrival on the island, so my early experiments with this unforgiving device resulted in a slew of regrettable bald areas on Michael's scalp. He was sometimes asked if he had a nasty fungal condition to account for these grotesque patches; but I was gratified that he was largely unaware of just how disfiguring they were, as most were fortuitously located on the back of his head.

Of course, I practised on our kids as well as him and, with time and experience, I gradually became safer and more proficient with scissors and shaver. Eventually, some of our neighbours even asked me to give them a trim, and I was happy to oblige as part of the give-and-take of island life.

Above the doorway of our lounge-room, as I snipped away at various heads of hair, I imagined a large curly pink sign in bright, bold letters advertising the name of my proposed establishment. The virtual words that flashed up in my mind's eye proudly proclaimed the motivation of my home-based 'salon,' suitably expressed by the shiny, sparkly title of:

'Shear Necessity!'

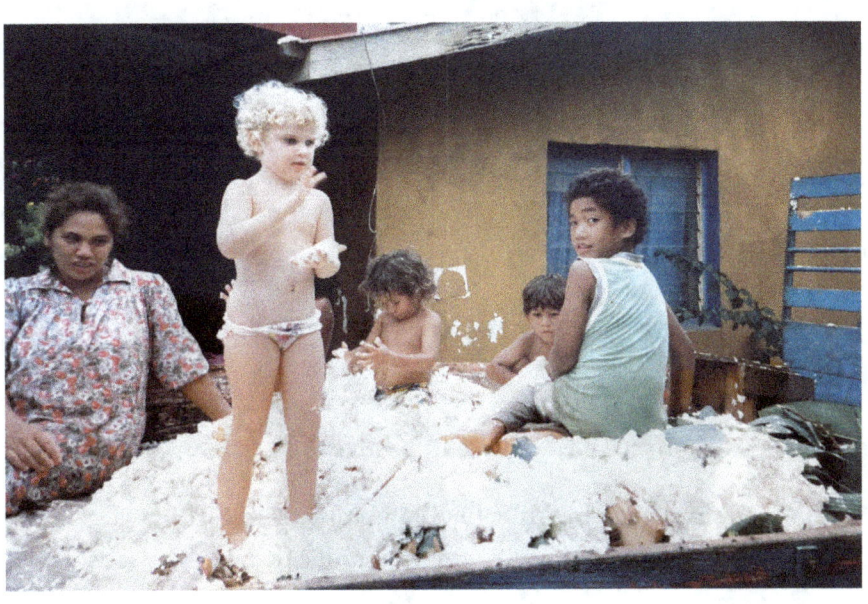

Rhiannon with local kids playing with arrowroot husks.

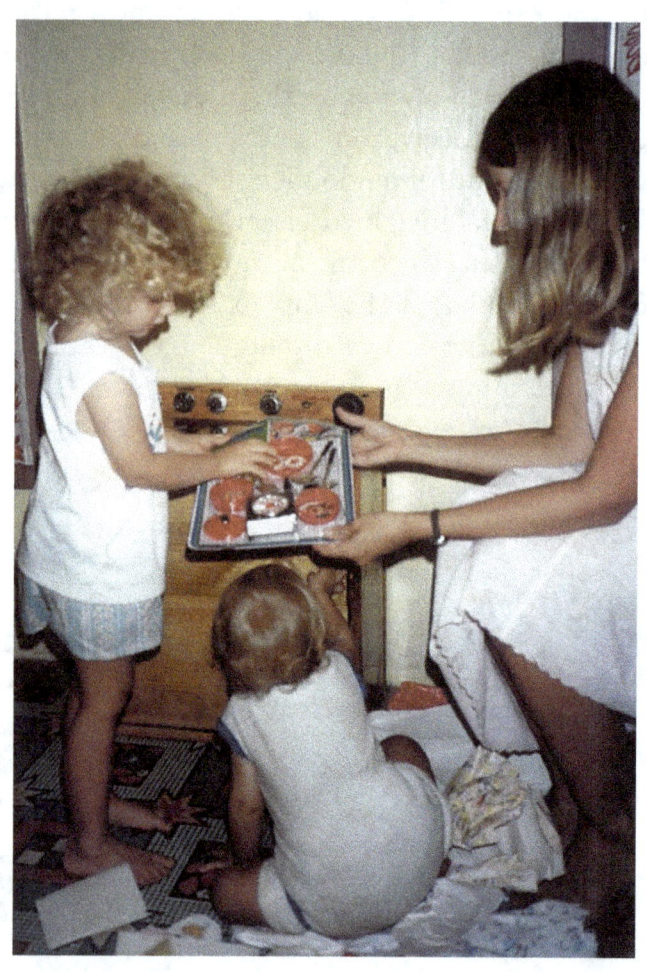

Stove made by Mike for Rhiannon's third birthday on 28/4/1988 with kids and Michele.

14 - Supplies

Shopping for food was an erratic undertaking on the island – we never knew when we set out for provisions whether we would come home flushed with success and eager to tuck into something rare and tasty, or else return empty-handed and despondent that the shops were all but empty once again. The latter was very discouraging – especially when the only fresh vegetable we had at home was a small tub of taro.

The main staples that were usually available were locally produced, including bananas, pawpaws, coconuts, fish and root vegetables such as arrowroot or *kumara*. Other foods were either seasonally grown (citrus, mangoes, avocados and some vegetables) or brought in by the supply ships. The imports were sold at two of the four small shops on the island. One of these stores sold hardware, household items and tinned foods; two shops were small bakeries; and another sold packaged, canned and frozen foods. Unfortunately, none of them sold fresh fruit or vegetables, and there were no markets on the island either.

Given the monopoly on prices and difficulties with supply,

food was expensive compared with Australian prices at the time: a dozen small eggs cost $5, an 800g chicken was $7, ice-cream was $7.50 for 2 litres, and cheese (that had invariably passed its New Zealand expiry date by months) was $8 for 500g – all in local currency or New Zealand dollars (NZD). In fact, it seemed to be a regular pattern for Kiwi suppliers to forward their expired stock to the Cooks to continue to make a profit. Nevertheless, regardless of the cost or age of these foodstuffs, we treasured them so much that we were happy to buy them whenever they were available. We also stored whatever we could in our tiny freezer, to make them last for as long as possible.

Midway through our first year on the island, there was a knock at the kitchen door and I answered it to find one of the hospital gardeners carrying a bucket of tomatoes in one hand and a large cabbage in the other.

'Hi Mrs Dr Browne,' he grinned, 'Dr Rua said you need this food so I bring some for you.'

I gave him a grateful smile: 'Oh, thank you so much Oatu, that's very kind of you. Did you grow them yourself?'

He carried the vegetables through the doorway and put them onto the kitchen bench.

'Yeah, in my garden,' he said, inclining his head modestly.

'I wish we could grow some like that too,' I replied; 'How do you stop the chooks and bugs from eating them all?'

He shrugged his massive shoulders, possibly not understanding the question or not knowing enough English to answer. He walked back towards the door, but I touched his arm and said: 'Please let me give you some money – we're very happy to pay you.'

I reached for my purse from the kitchen drawer, but he backed out of the doorway, shaking his head in horror, as though I'd just slapped him in the face.

'No, no, all good,' he insisted. He walked back to the hospital ambulance that was parked in the driveway.

'I'll make you some cake,' I called out, and he nodded and smiled as he started the engine and drove off.

'Who was that?' asked Mike, as he came into the kitchen and put on the kettle.

I got out some mugs. 'Oatu dropped in some fresh vegetables. I offered to pay him, but he flat-out refused. It's tricky isn't it?'

'Yes, I know what you mean.' Mike picked up a tomato from the bucket and began to make some sandwiches with it for lunch. 'It's nice of them to give us their home-grown stuff, but then when we run out, it feels really rude to ask for more.'

'Exactly.' I filled the tea-pot with boiling water. 'He said Dr Rua had asked him to bring it over for us, which was really kind of him. But it's such a shame that we can't get fresh veggies in the shops – I'd much rather just buy what we want whenever we need it, and not feel like we're expecting the locals to give us their food. After all, they've got their own families to feed.'

'Mm. I also wish our own garden was more productive – then we wouldn't need to ask,' Mike added, with a dispirited frown; 'The plan was that we'd be eating our own veggies by now, especially with the cooler weather lately, but that's certainly not the case.'

'Yeah – it's such a pain. I asked Oatu how his crops survived the chooks and bugs, but he didn't seem to know what I meant. Looks like his feral-proofing techniques will remain a secret.'

I lifted Thomas into his high-chair and placed a sandwich in front of him.

Mike grinned. 'Well, one thing's not a secret, that's for sure – we'll soon be making some more cakes again. It's always acceptable currency in this part of the world.'

The shops on Aitutaki were very dependent on supply boats to maintain their stock, and they arrived every four to six weeks. However, a significant difficulty with accessing the island was that, although the passage through the reef was ten metres wide, it was only two metres deep, even at high tide. This meant that any vessel with a draught deeper than a medium-sized motorboat had to anchor outside the lagoon – and that included the supply ships too. Mooring in the open seas exposed them to significant winds and swells, making it hard to load or unload supplies.

The only way that items could reach the island was by shifting them from the supply vessels onto a barge that was about eight by four metres, and hauling it with a tugboat through the reef passage to port. However, if there were storms at the time of the ship's arrival, attempts would be made to move the stock for about two days, but if this was unsuccessful, the vessel would have to progress onto its next port, leaving us all empty-handed and downhearted in its wake.

'Ok kids, let's go and do the shopping,' I called out, and they looked up from their Duplo creations on the lounge-room floor.

Rhiannon shoved her plastic building aside. 'Great! I hope we can get Rice Bubbles today – and maybe even some biscuits.'

She looked at me expectantly and I smiled. 'Well, we'll see what they've got. I heard the supply boat came in yesterday, so maybe it brought some nice things to eat.'

We climbed into the car and drove into 'town'. The shop most likely to have our preferred staples was at the end of the short main road, so I parked out the front and unbuckled the kids from their car-seats. But all was subdued when we went inside and the bored shop girl was flicking through an islander newspaper. We looked around at the shelves and soon realised that there were no dairy products or household items, and no dried, tinned, packaged or frozen foods either. In fact, the shop was even more empty than the last time we'd come in.

'Where's all the food gone?' Rhiannon wailed and the girl at the checkout looked up.

'The seas were too rough to load the barge – same as last month. You could try again in four or six weeks.' She shrugged dismissively and returned to her reading.

I crouched down in front of the kids who were both sobbing by now. 'I'm sorry, you two. Looks like the boat couldn't bring the food we wanted this time. We'll have to manage with what we've got at home for now.'

I found it hard not to weep myself. Our supplies of many things were already pathetically low, so meals in the weeks ahead were going to require considerable ingenuity. Maybe someone might drop in a fish or some home-grown veg – or an invitation to a *kaikai* – now that would be helpful...

Rhiannon's cries grew louder and Thomas followed suit, drawing my attention back to the present moment. I hugged them both then stood up to shepherd them outside.

'I think there might be some chocolate at home,' I said as I did up their car-seats, 'I've been saving it for a while now, but I think we could try to find it when we get home, huh?'

They sniffled and I wiped their faces. 'Let's drive back and take a look.'

I was thankful that some of our visitors had brought over our favourite treats, and I kept them hidden away in case of emergencies. It was definitely time to open one of these today.

Desperate times called for desperate measures...

We climbed back into the car to go in search of comfort food once again. As we drove past the wharf, I noticed some of the local men putting boxes of bananas onto the back of their trucks. Sadly, their latest banana harvest wasn't able to reach the supply ship either, so now it would all be wasted. Feeling sorry for them, I gave a friendly wave, and they nodded back in a disheartened fashion.

Supply boat issues affected the Māori much more seriously than us, due to past political and economic decisions. Apparently since the 1960s, local governments had decided that it would be best for individual islands within the Cooks to specialise in cultivating a particular tropical crop, a plan that was intended to maximise export earnings for each island. Rarotonga and Aitutaki mainly grew bananas; Penrhyn and Rakahanga produced copra; Manihiki cultured trochus shells that contained mother of pearl or *padua*; and Mangaia and Atiu cultivated pineapples and citrus.

Unfortunately, Cyclone Sally had not only damaged many houses on Aitutaki in January 1987, it had also wiped out many of the banana plantations, along with the packing sheds at the wharf and the banana drying factory nearby. The industry was only just beginning to recover a year or so later, so several days before a supply boat was due to arrive, the Māori harvested large stalks of bananas, sprayed them and boxed them up ready for sale.

However, a vital link in the export chain was missing: there was no system of refrigerated storage at the port. Tragically therefore, if the barge couldn't reach the supply boat and transfer its stock, the entire harvested crop would be wasted. There was no other means of selling the fruit, even though it was likely that *papa'as*, locals and tourists would have purchased at least some of it, if it had been placed in the local shops. Sadly, that didn't happen at the time though, so the picked bananas were simply fed to the pigs and the islanders earned nothing for all their labour. It was truly heart-breaking to see them looking so wretched.

Our own banana supply was usually maintained by the hospital groundsmen, or others who noticed when they rode past that our stock had dropped to a paltry 75kg or so. Then they added further stalks to those hanging from our carport roof and removed the over-ripe ones. Hearing about our vast banana reserves, my parents had posted us a book called: '101 Ways with Bananas' – it proved to be a valuable tome for a surprising variety of sweet and savoury recipes.

Local growers urged us to come and collect our own bananas from their farms, on the rare occasions when we needed to restock ourselves. Mike would take the kids on these excursions, and Thomas had a favourite outfit, his 'banana shorts,' that he liked to wear to collect the hefty stalks. They all enjoyed these small adventures and the connection with the friendly local farmers and their families.

Once again, we would have been happy to buy their fruit, but this was anathema to the islanders. Perhaps in part, it was due to them valuing the free medical care and kitchen consultations that we provided, and they wanted to express their gratitude in the way they knew best. We had already learned that, in Māori culture, positive sentiments or social affirmation of any kind almost invariably involved the giving and receiving of food, and true to form, this was usually done with a generosity that bordered on the bizarre!

Occasionally, we received medical supplies from erratic donations from various hospitals, aid organisations or defence forces. If there had been a recent visit to the island from New Zealand or Australian armed services, they would often leave behind their unused stock, which came in very handy. When unpacking one such box of second-hand materials, we came across some bandages that were packed by the US Army in May 1957 – before either of us was even born – and definitely a record for the age of our supplies!

One quiet afternoon, our family headed up to the hospital to clean up the dispensary and do the usual monthly repackaging of medications into our hand-made envelopes. But as we walked in, I noticed that the shelves were looking much more barren than usual.

'Where are all the bandages, plasters and crutches?' I asked.

Mike frowned and opened a few drawers and cupboards where any overflow could have been stored. 'I don't know. I knew we were running low on some things, but it looks like we've pretty much run out.'

'We had better check the last list that we sent to Raro – I'm sure we wouldn't have forgotten to put those on the order-sheet,' I added.

He went to our clinic room, rummaged through the desk drawer and found our spare copy.

'No, we didn't forget – look,' he said as he returned and passed it to me.

Sure enough, we had ordered them all, along with numerous other regular supplies: IV fluids, local anaesthetics, suture materials, dressings and medications. But next to many of the items on the return list, there were initials from the Raro dispensary stating: 'Not supplied' or comments that less than half of our requested order had been sent through.

Like the island's food, our regular hospital stock was reliant on the supply boats; but there were additional complexities in the system that made this process especially convoluted. During our time at Raro Hospital, we had noted the abundance of medical supplies there, and had been instructed in the paperwork necessary to have them delivered to us on each supply vessel. It seemed logical enough: we sent a list to Raro Hospital Pharmacy specifying exactly what we needed, and they packaged up these items ready for the next boat, in order to reach us in a prompt and orderly way.

Simple.

But no – this apparently straight-forward process stalled with monotonous regularity, creating considerable difficulties for us and many others on the island.

'We had better do a stock-take,' I said, starting to feel queasy at the thought of how we were going to be able to treat our patients when so few of the essential items were available.

Three-year-old Rhiannon clambered onto the bench where she usually helped to count out the pills. She and I checked the oral preparations, while Mike did the other stock, and one-year-old Thomas tore out pages from the dusty magazines on the floor.

'How did you go?' I asked Mike a short time later.

He shook his head. 'We've barely got enough here to last for another fortnight and I don't think there's another boat due for at least a month. What about you two?'

'Well, we've completely run out of cough syrup and inhalers, and we've only got about one or two courses of pills for hypertension, diabetes or contraception.'

'And we've got twenty-three of this kind.' Rhiannon held up the tray of Amoxicillin capsules that she had just counted out.

'Thanks love,' I said, 'But they're all going to be used up in no time.'

'I'll have to ring the Raro Hospital dispensary first thing on Monday,' Mike said, moving aside a pile of old journals from Thomas, so they weren't all decimated; 'I'll see if they can get a wriggle on.'

However, his phone call was met with an indignant reaction by the thorny Pharmacy manager at Raro Hospital, who claimed that our requested stock had either been supplied, or would be on the next boat, and denying that there were any shortages. Attempts to repudiate his statements went nowhere, so we elected to wait for the supply ship that was due in another four weeks.

In the meantime, to add insult to injury, we received a telegram from the Raro dispensary a week later instructing us and every other outer island in the Cooks to return all our oral contraceptives to them, despite the manager's previous assertions that there was no shortfall in their supplies. We snorted in disgust at this galling request and accidentally 'lost' the telegram into the nearest bin.

When the next supply ship arrived, we were disappointed to discover that, yet again, it had brought only a meagre proportion of our requested items. As it happened, this situation coincided with the approach of Health Week on Aitutaki – an annual event during which we were supposed to emphasise the importance of preventive health, early interventions, and encouraging the locals to take their prescribed medications regularly. *Difficult to do if we don't even have their tablets in our dispensary,* I reflected ruefully. The motto for Health Week at that time was: 'Let's talk Health!'

Mike wrote a letter to the Director General of Health stating that we were now critically depleted in our essential dispensary items. He included a copy of our order form that the Raro Pharmacy had returned to us with its minimal stock that stated

'Not supplied' next to almost every entry.

Mike concluded his letter to the Director with the following words: *The irony of 'Health Week' approaching with our dispensary shelves nearly empty has not been missed by the staff or the general community, and I hope our hospital will be in a healthier state by the time it is celebrated. Perhaps I could suggest a slight modification to the motto for the occasion to state more appropriately: "Less talk Health!"*

A few days after Health Week had come and gone, Mike paced angrily around the dining-room when he came home for lunch. 'Can you believe it? Our entire antibiotic supply consists of *six* Bactrim tablets.'

'*What?*'

'But that's the *good* news,' he added fiercely, 'It's the only stock we have of *anything!* Apart from those, the dispensary is *completely empty*: no crutches, bandages, suture materials, plasters, IV fluids, medications – *nothing!*'

I stared at him with horror. 'Oh no – what on earth are we going to do now?'

'I've tried to work out some ideas,' he replied, shaking his head, 'But the only one that makes any sense is to contact the Director General of Health, and tell him that we'll have to close the hospital until we get the resources to actually treat our patients. Look, the locals are amazing – much more accepting than anyone in Australia would be under these conditions – but this is just *ridiculous.*'

That afternoon, Mike sent a telegram to the Director stating: '*Dispensary resources critically low, with NO essential medications or supplies left. Please see previous order form for details. Unless rectified immediately, will have no option but to close Aitutaki Hospital forthwith.*'

The Director rang back later that day in a state of high

dudgeon. He seemed to consider Mike's ultimatum about closing the hospital as an absurd over-reaction, despite Mike pointing out that our dispensary was now completely empty, the last few antibiotic tablets having been dispensed earlier that day. Eventually, however, the Director agreed to send the vital supplies to us urgently.

Mike slammed the phone down. 'Well – let's see what happens now. I told him the last order form has the exact list of everything we need, and he said he'd be airlifting it all here tomorrow morning on a commercial flight.'

I shook my head in disbelief at such a terrible waste of resources. 'Just imagine what that'll cost the Health Department – and all because someone in Raro Hospital can't be bothered to find the stuff and send it through to us by boat in good time.'

Whenever these kinds of scenarios occurred, we oscillated between teeth-grinding frustration *(Why should this arrangement be so difficult?)* and helpless resignation *(If this is the way they want to do things, then we should just let them get on with it. This is their health system, so it's not our job to tell them what to do...).*

The following day, at appalling expense, a domestic flight arrived with eight large cylinders of oxygen (that we hadn't requested); massive crates of IV fluids (twelve times the volume that we had asked for); and several large boxes of medications that bore little resemblance to the forwarded request forms. The suspensions of our two ambulances groaned under the weight of all these supplies, as they transported multiple loads from the airport to the hospital, while the staff chattered in excitement at the unfolding drama.

It was a relief to have some stock in the dispensary at last. But since the brands and dosages of many drugs were not what we had requested, we had to spend the ensuing months trying to re-adjust our patients' medications to whatever we'd received that approximated their previous regimes. It was tedious work, and especially irritating when we had been told that Raro was well-stocked in the specific products that we had ordered.

Sometimes tourists we met around Aitutaki told us that we lived in paradise, and how they envied us for what they imagined to be our delightful and relaxed way of life. But with situations such as these, it felt like a hellish experience to be *papa'as* trapped on a tiny atoll in the middle of nowhere, in an incompetent and apathetic supply system, where we were expected to provide quality medical care in an empty hospital building.

Sanity required an exquisitely balanced combination of calm thinking that approached nirvanic detachment, slow measured mindful breathing, and a sense of humour that bordered on mania at the quixotic nature of life on the island.

Suffice to say: some days were definitely better than others.

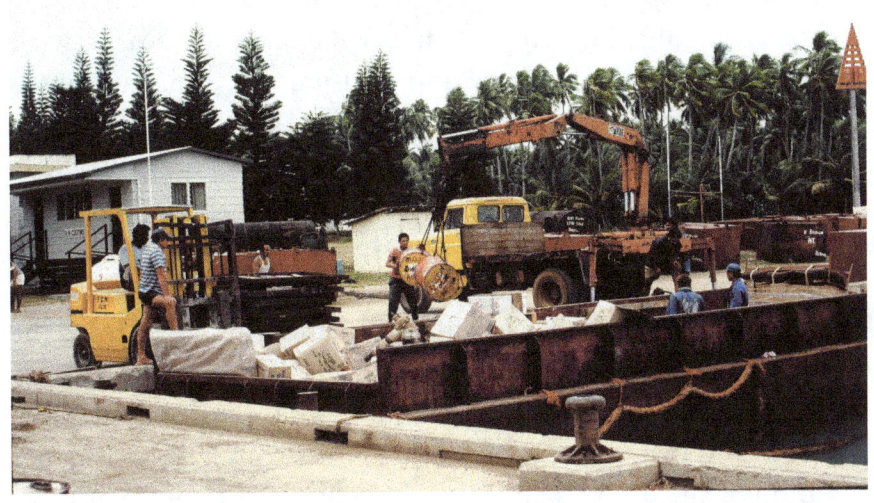

Crane and barge used to transport supplies onto the island.

15 – Mosquito Management

Several months after our arrival on Aitutaki, Moana, one of the Public Health officers, came up to Outpatients at the end of the morning. He informed Mike that on the following day, they needed him to assist the Public Health team in a mosquito eradication programme. Mike had no idea of what exactly this task would entail and as usual, no explanation was forthcoming from the laconic islander; but he packed an ample lunch that evening to take with him, just to cover the most likely contingencies.

The Public Health officers and hospital groundsmen collected him on the all-purpose ambulance at dawn and they travelled to the edge of the mainland. Climbing down from the ute, they stood together to begin the day's activities with their familiar ritual of prayer. Rima, one of the gardeners, did the honours and his supplications seemed to encompass many issues – although since it was all in Māori, Mike had to guess at most of the content. Touched by their obvious sincerity though, he watched as several of the men wiped tears from their eyes as the intercessions concluded.

The group then swung into action by tossing a large pile of equipment into a motorboat, climbing aboard and navigating to a nearby *motu*. Moana distributed machetes and the men hacked their way to the centre of the small islet until they came across a suspected mosquito breeding area. Rima then produced a further pile of spades, axes and crowbars so that the men could clear the plant-life and sand away from the opening of a mangrove swamp and improve its drainage into the lagoon.

The sultry heat was clammy in the dense vegetation, and menacing mosquitoes hovered around the men as they laboured on, with only an occasional sharp instruction barked by one of the leaders. The thudding of heavy tools was muffled in the thick suffocating air and sweat poured from their glistening bodies.

As he tried to keep up with the others, Mike wondered why he'd been asked to join the team for the day's pursuits. After all, he knew as much as any Canberra GP about the Polynesian mosquito and effective strategies to curb its breeding rates – so he wasn't confident that he had a lot to contribute, either academically or manually. Nevertheless, he resolved to give it his best shot, since it was a day away from the office and he hoped he could learn something of value.

Some hours and considerable efforts later, the team had created a channel that was about fifteen metres long, a metre wide and half a metre deep, to direct the marshy water from the mangrove swamp into the lagoon. Mike stopped digging to take another hefty gulp from his water bottle and view the outcome of their labours.

'Hey, Moana,' he called out, 'Has anyone thought of getting some heavy-duty machinery down here to tackle this drainage problem?'

Moana gave him a wary eye. 'What kind of machines?'

'Well, you could use the harbour barge to transport one of the big front-end loaders from the mainland to this *motu*. That way some serious excavation could be done – and much faster than us, too.'

The team paused and leant on their spades to listen to this dialogue.

Moana frowned in horror. 'No, doctor – if we did that, it would make this a Public *Works* Project. *We* have to do the digging so that it's a Public *Health* Project.' His expression turned from one of dismay into a scowl of frank distaste. 'We couldn't use *machines.*'

'Oh, I see,' Mike said, although he didn't really. The rest of the men simply nodded and got back to their shovelling.

Mike was amused that such a fierce demarcation dispute could exist between two such small departments on this usually indolent island. At least Moana's explanation provided a clue as to why Mike had been requested to attend: in the eyes of the islanders, he served as a mascot for the Health Department to ensure that the Public Works Department kept their distance from this assignment, and couldn't receive the credit for any possible successes, no matter how unlikely.

As the sun climbed to its penetrating zenith, Rima called time for lunch. It seemed an incongruous thing to do, since there was no food in evidence at all, apart from Mike's packet of sandwiches. The Māori responded with disparaging sneers when Mike pulled them out of his backpack and he watched to see how they intended to feed themselves.

With no apparent organisation, two groundsmen found some long sticks, sharpened them with their machetes, wandered along the beach and skilfully speared five large trevally. Elsewhere, another worker climbed a tree, returning with three substantial breadfruits, and another scaled palms to toss down a pile of *nu*. Meanwhile Moana and Rima gathered rocks and shells, prepared a fire to heat them, and laid the whole fish and breadfruit on top until everything was cooked to perfection.

Voilà – Real Man Food!

Setting aside his packed lunch that was now embarrassingly redundant, Mike joined in with the others and relished the delicious meal and sense of camaraderie that followed. It was a moment to savour – sitting on this unspoiled shady beach and eating a natural repast with these skilful hunter-gatherers, while listening to their quiet banter – what could be better?

Of course, lunch was followed by an obligatory communal nap for an hour or two, while the cool sea breeze caressed their weary bodies.

By the time they returned to their worksite a few hours later, the gentle waves of the incoming tide had all but obliterated the former channel, as the fine white sand of the beach rapidly returned to its usual pristine position. None of the Public Health team seemed overly concerned by this outcome. Perhaps a boys' day out on the *motu* with their own *kaikai* was the real point of the exercise after all…

Later in the afternoon, Rima ordered them to collect their tools and they all piled into the boat, then the ambulance for the trip back home. As they travelled along, Mike thought that perhaps it was time he made a *papa'a* contribution to this deeply mystifying process.

'Has anyone suggested some more ways to help with the problem of the mosquitoes?' he asked.

The men considered this quietly for a while and then Moana spoke up.

'Yeah, well a few years ago, the World Health Organisation sent some *papa'as* to Raro and Aitutaki. They come from some different countries round the world to check the mosquitoes.

They even do photos and make maps from aeroplanes to think up good ideas to help us,' he added.

'How long were they here?' Mike asked. The thorough process had him intrigued.

'I think about three or four months altogether,' Moana replied; 'They write up two big folders with all the things they think when they finish.'

The other men, who had listened in, resumed their quiet dozy state as the ambulance swayed along the bush track.

Mike had the feeling that there were disturbing gaps in the transfer of this information. 'Well, where are the reports now?'

'They give a copy to Raro and one for our hospital too,' Moana concluded, implying that that was the end of the matter.

The men nodded and silence descended once again.

'Well, what did they say in the reports?' Mike couldn't help but ask.

'Ah, we don't know,' Moana replied reluctantly, as though the topic was somehow taboo; 'We can't really understand it.' His usual confidence appeared to dissolve as he stared at the floor of the ute.

'But why not?' Mike persisted. He reasoned that *some* islanders in the health or political system would have been sufficiently motivated to read these important documents, produced after so much effort and expense – and then there was the necessity of implementing their recommendations, of course…

Moana fixed his gaze moodily at the bumpy track as they all lurched with the vehicle. After an uncomfortable pause, he finally said, 'Well, we just can't read it.'

'Well, why ever not?' Mike enquired, frustrated by the evasive and convoluted replies.

Moana looked at Mike and slowly, with a resigned shrug of

his huge shoulders, added in a subdued monotone: 'You see, the report – yeah, well everything – it was all written in French.'

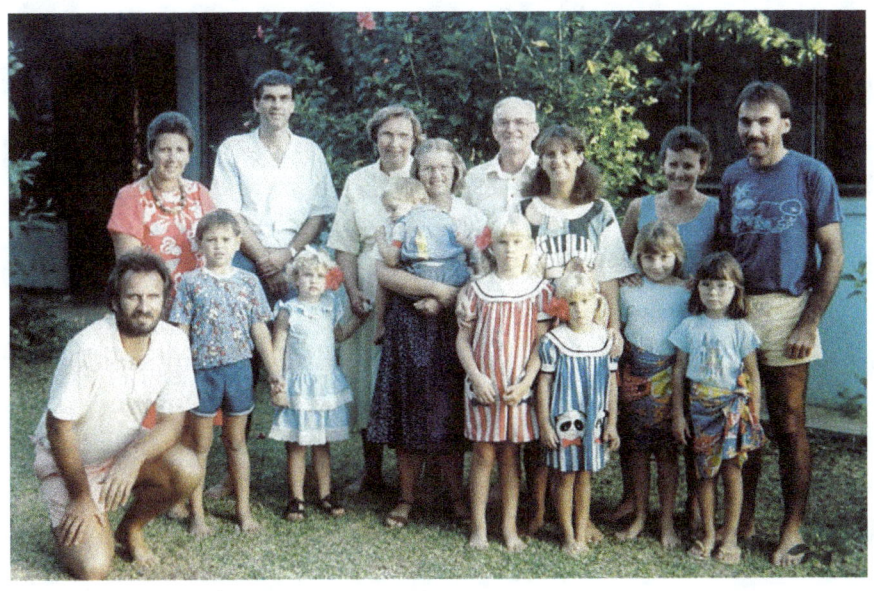

Friends & neighbours in mid-1989.
L>R Back row: Margaret, Mike, Rachel, Sam, Judi F, Roger F.
Middle row: RB, Anton, Rhiannon, Michele holding Thomas, JB, Gemma F, Hannah F.
Front row: MB, SB. (RB, JB, MB & SB – AVA neighbours. JF, RF, GF & HF – the Files, a Kiwi family from across the road.)

16 – Families

A frantic knock at the kitchen door disturbed our quiet evening, and I answered it to find a man holding a limp ashen two-year-old in his arms. Her sunken eyes rolled backwards in their sockets and her shrivelled skin stretched over her flaccid limbs.

I gave a horrified gasp. 'Mike – quick, *quick* – this kid looks like she's about to die.'

He ran into the kitchen and the Māori father stared at both of us with beseeching eyes, too frightened to say a word.

'Come with me,' Mike said to the man, grabbing the car keys, 'We'll drive straight to the hospital in my car.'

They disappeared through the doorway and the car revved out of the driveway.

'We need IV fluids as fast as possible,' Mike said to the nurse who met them in the hospital ward after hearing the car doors slam. She hurried to get the necessary equipment as Mike took the young girl from her father and placed her gently on the operating theatre bed.

'What happened?' Mike said, trying to pay attention to the father while he felt for her rapid pulse rate. He also noted that her tongue was bone dry.

'She's been throwing up and having runny poohs for two days,' the father replied.

'Has she been able to drink much today?' Mike asked as the nurse returned with the giving sets and fluids. He inserted a cannula into each arm and adjusted both IVs to maximal speed.

'Not much I think.' The islander spread his hands in a helpless gesture. 'My wife's family been looking after her, but a few kids been sick at the same time. They don't think she's thirsty, she only drink a bit. She been sleeping a lot – maybe too much…' A sob choked off any further words.

Other relatives gradually arrived and stood around the room in silent anguish. The unconscious child stirred a deep sense of dread within them all.

Unfortunately, despite Mike's best efforts, the little girl died within several hours from severe dehydration and secondary organ failure.

'I'm so sorry,' he said to the grieving parents afterwards, 'She was just too far gone by the time we started the fluids.'

He felt a miserable jumble of trauma at the loss of such a young child while under his care, distress for the family, and yet profound frustration that she may have survived had her parents sought help sooner. As there were no morgue facilities available on the island, she was buried the next afternoon, alongside too many other small plots in the family grave-site.

This tragic story was repeated several times during our posting, when other children died from conditions that may have been treatable had they been brought to the hospital earlier. These scenarios exposed the down-side of the extended family arrangement of islander society, where multiple carers came and went, without noting or passing on their concerns to one another. Of course, the same situation can also occur in any community in which adults fail to respond promptly enough to serious illness in their kids, with the same deadly results.

~

Before we arrived in the Cooks, I had believed that bonding between mothers and their babies was mostly due to emotional and hormonal changes during and after pregnancy, leading to the maternal drive to nurture their young. According to my reading and experience, this instinct appeared to supersede time, place and culture. But I later discovered that my understanding was far from accurate when it came to Māori practices.

The new Women's Health Clinic expanded my awareness of the complexities of islander family structure. Many of the older mamas had lost babies due to the exceptionally high infant mortality rates that had existed several decades earlier, but others had 'lost' babies in other ways. A particular interview remains firmly etched in my memory.

'So Mama Toru, how many pregnancies have you had?' I enquired of the woman at her clinic visit.

'Four babies,' the mama replied.

'How old are they now?'

'Oh, I think maybe the oldest is twelve and youngest is seven.' She frowned in concentration, as if recalling the details was difficult.

'How many of them live with you now?'

'Ah – *those* ones?' she asked, sounding puzzled.

'Yes, the ones that you gave birth to,' I confirmed.

'No, none of *those* ones,' Mama Toru said pragmatically.

'Where are they now?' I persisted.

'Oh well, oldest is with my first man's mother, next one's with my mother, next one –' she paused for a moment, 'Oh yes, she's with my sister in Raro and youngest lives in New Zealand with my cousin.'

'Right. So how many children live in your house now?' I'd learnt that I had to ask *all* the questions.

'Ah, four kids live in my house with me,' she said, as though this were somehow self-evident.

'Who had those kids, *their* mamas? And how old are they?' She was starting to get fed up, so I knew I had to speed up or miss the moment.

'Oldest one is ten and next one is eight – they come from my brother in Mauke. Next one is six – she come from my other sister in Raro, and youngest kid is five – he from my cousin in Vaipae.'

'OK – so let's just check this again: you had four babies, but they all live somewhere else?' I asked and the mama nodded slowly; 'And now you have four more kids from other people in your family, who *you* look after at your place?'

'Ah, yeah,' she beamed. We had finally got it sorted.

~

Islander children were acquired or given away with remarkable frequency and informality compared with the norm in western societies, and infants were often raised by the extended family rather than their own biological parents. Often the firstborn was given to grandparents to be raised, but then further offspring could also be 'claimed' by other relatives, with or without much input from their birth mothers. These loosely acquired extras were called 'feeding children.'

In some ways, this *avant-garde* approach to parenthood

seemed to work quite well – at least every child in Māori society had *someone* who was willing to raise them and was often related to them, thus providing a wider sense of family. It also obviated our problematic western system of trying to find foster homes or adoptive parents for vulnerable children.

But Māori traditions around family life had their own challenges too. In previous generations, 'feeding children' may not have lived with their own parents, but they would have lived near them on the same island and even in the same village. Once modern travel intervened however, children could be moved to more remote islands, or other countries, with the potential to seriously disrupt their sense of identity, belonging and cultural background.

I found it all very confronting.

The giving away of children was something we witnessed on multiple occasions during our posting. Māori families from overseas would visit their relatives on the island and sometimes the Aitutakians became fond of one of their visitors' children. Discussions would then occur where the locals asked if they could keep a youngster when the rest of the family returned home. If the visitors were agreeable, the child was left in the care of their islander family, sometimes for long periods or even indefinitely.

I tried to imagine how devastating this arrangement could be for the young child involved. It seemed highly likely that losing contact with all the familiar people in their world, and having them replaced by complete strangers, must have caused them serious trauma. In fact, I have never been able to get my head or my heart around how this cultural practice played out for the little ones involved, as well as for their siblings and parents. Of course, islanders viewed this system as normal and didn't consider that it could be problematic. But I believed (possibly inaccurately) that the impact would surely be profound and long term, just as it has been in many other 'stolen children' scenarios around the world.

Variations on the child-swapping arrangements also occurred. I vividly remember seeing the reverse scenario unfolding for my cleaner-cum-nurse friend, Tiare. Although she had been born in Aitutaki, she had spent some of her teen years in New Zealand, so she was more westernised in her attitudes than many other young Māori women.

'Tell me about your kids,' I said to her one afternoon as we shared a quiet cuppa after the women's clinic had finished.

Tiare smiled warmly. 'My first one is a girl, like yours, and she's two and a half now.'

I nodded and asked, 'So who looks after her when you're at work?'

Tiare frowned. 'She lives with my parents-in-law – but not just when I work – all the time.'

'Oh, how did that happen?' I said, trying not to sound as surprised as I felt.

'Well, when she was born, they said they wanted to have her, cos they wanted another girl.' I could hear the strain in her voice and her discomfort with the situation.

'Ah – so you couldn't just say that you wanted to keep her, then?' I asked, feeling a rising sense of disquiet.

'No. My husband said we had to give her to them, or there'd be family trouble.' Tears gathered in her eyes and she rubbed her face with the backs of her hands. 'But they just live in Ureia, the next village, so I can see her quite a lot.'

I nodded slowly. 'Well, that's good. And do you have any other kids?'

'Yes, just one, a boy. He's called Taku – in Māori that means 'Mine' because he will stay with me.' Now her tears were joyful ones. 'Mr Dr Browne delivered him – he's five months old now, and I still breastfeed him myself.'

Her accomplishment was a source of gentle pride and we smiled together.

'Well done! You must bring him in one day so I can meet him,' I said and she nodded keenly as we gathered up our cups and headed to the staffroom.

Several days later, Tiare arrived at the hospital with her son, a bonny boy who clearly gave her enormous delight. We chatted about Taku and his progress, and she showed him off to her workmates. All islanders love babies – I had previously noticed that even teenage boys were comfortable holding young ones and watching out for them. The staff clucked over Taku and we all had a cuddle of him before his mother took him home.

A few months later when I saw Tiare at work, I asked her how Taku was going. I was sorry to see her eyes quickly filling with tears.

'What's happened?' I said, fearing that he'd developed a serious illness.

'Some relatives came over to visit from New Zealand a few weeks ago,' she began, trembling a little; 'They're my husband's family and they're staying with his parents for a while.'

'Yes,' I coaxed, not seeing anything of immediate concern.

Her voice faltered: 'Well, they said they really like Taku and they want to take him back to New Zealand with them, when they go home.'

A sense of panic rose up in me as comprehension dawned. 'Oh, gosh. How many weeks would he be going for? Just a short visit?'

'I don't know cos they won't say. Maybe he'll have to stay with them for a long time…' Her voice was choked with grief.

I was aghast, imagining how I'd feel if someone wanted to

take either of my children away from me, even briefly, let alone to another country and indefinitely. Not only had she 'lost' her daughter, but now her son was being taken away, and much further afield too.

'Can't you just say "No"?' I asked rather forcefully.

'But they'll be upset and angry with me.' She gave a shrug of helpless misery and dissolved into tears.

That argument didn't hold much weight with me, but clearly in her culture, refusing to give up your child when someone asked you nicely was simply not the done thing – apparently, it could be construed as causing major family strife.

So what? I was thinking as fierce maternal rage coursed through my being.

Tiare told me how she'd felt ignored and overwhelmed by the pressure she was under. She rocked back and forth and, as we talked about it further, we hugged and cried together in mutual distress.

About a month later, when I asked her how things had worked out, the tears flowed down her face again. She told me that, during the previous week, when the Kiwi family had boarded the Cook Island Air flight for home, they had proudly carried her young son back to New Zealand with them, into an unknown future for all concerned. Meanwhile, his mother had desperately waved and wept for her Taku at the airport railing, her empty arms hugging her swollen breasts in lonely aching sorrow.

~

Before my arrival, I had naïvely imagined that islander women would nurse their babies for long periods, so I was unprepared for the discovery that breastfeeding was often quite an abbreviated affair amongst the local mamas. It seemed that they frequently wanted to leave their infants with others, in addition to giving them away altogether, and therefore nursing was widely regarded as an inconvenience by many of them.

I had taken Thomas with me to the *Tivaevae* group one afternoon when he was twelve months old. As we sat in a circle on the floor of the village hall to sew together, he breastfed voraciously as usual and the mamas took the opportunity to ask me some medical questions.

'Hey Mrs Dr Browne,' one mama asked, 'Can I feed my boy some baked beans now?'

'How old is he?' I asked, noting that the baby beside her on a rug still looked very young.

'He's six weeks already – he's getting big.' She smiled proudly at her son and I knew I had to give my opinion carefully.

'Yes, he *is* growing well. But he's not very old and his body can't handle baked beans yet. He could get quite sick in his belly.'

'What about Weetbix?' asked another mother as she cradled her infant daughter in her lap while sewing a cushion cover.

'Same thing, I'm afraid. Babies can't eat that sort of food until they're about six months old.'

Another one tried, with confident authority: 'But Milo is good, huh?'

'No, not yet,' I confirmed, 'It's got lots of sugar in it and the young ones can't digest it properly till they're about one year old. It's better just to breastfeed for as long as you can.'

Several of the young women muttered resentfully and I thought I should give a little more detail. 'Back in my hometown we say: "Breast is best" and it's true. Breastmilk has all that babies need for the first six months at least, and most of what they need for twelve months or more.'

Another mama couldn't keep the sullen edge out of her

voice. 'But then you can't leave your *pepe* with someone else.'

'Yes, I know. But really, babies are only little for a short time and feeding them yourself for as long as you can keeps them healthy – it prevents many belly bugs and other infections.' I lifted Thomas to switch him to the other side and tried to give a more enticing ring to my sales pitch: 'And the good news is that you don't need to make up bottles or buy milk powder, so it saves you time and money, too.'

The mamas smiled at my words and shook their heads in disbelief.

'Ah, but you don't know about our island ways,' said one of them patronisingly; 'Your kind of feeding is just an old *papa'a* custom, huh?'

They all laughed uproariously at their own joke and pointed at Thomas as he peered back at them from his firmly attached position. I shook my head with a sad sense of defeat.

Their comments felt like the ultimate irony to me.

~

The curious attitudes of islanders to breastfeeding, family life and parenting continued to challenge Mike and me throughout our stay, and one memorable occasion crystallised some of these puzzling sentiments for both of us.

Yet again, the familiar revving of the ambulance sounded from our driveway late one afternoon.

'Uh-ohh, ambliance,' said eighteen-month-old Thomas, shaking his head philosophically. Running into the dining-room, he dragged Mike's work-bag across the floor towards the kitchen, calling out: 'Patient, patient!'

'Thanks mate.' Mike picked up his bag and tousled Thomas' hair affectionately as he headed out the door.

'Mama having *pepe*,' said the driver as Mike climbed into the ute.

A local woman was in labour and he arrived just in time to deliver a healthy little boy. Mike has always been very keen on babies – it's got a lot to do with why we ended up having four of our own, I think. So he cooed and clucked over this newborn, while the midwives cleaned up after the delivery.

'Hey Mama, here's your fine new son,' Mike said, holding him up for his mother to see, 'How about you put him on the breast for his first feed?'

But the woman laughed and waved her hands disparagingly, saying, 'No, no – I told my sister she could have this one if it was a boy – so he'll be on the next boat to Pukapuka.'

This was one of the northernmost islands in the Cooks, and a distance of about fourteen hundred kilometres from Aitutaki. It was extraordinarily remote at this time, with supply ships visiting only once every six months and no runway at all for planes to land. It seemed to us that being sent to Pukapuka was somewhat akin to being transported to a penal colony on the far side of the globe.

'But don't you want to breastfeed him till then?' Mike asked, trying to coax some semblance of bonding between mama and *pepe*.

She dismissed the idea with another wave of her hands, 'No, he'll only get used to it. Better he have bottle-milk or Milo till then.'

Mike was still trying to process the baby's future, in light of his mother's perplexing statements. 'But how often will you see him if he lives all the way up there?'

The mama laughed heartily again, 'Ah, I don't know – maybe never!'

Mike cradled the newborn against his chest and gazed at the

beautiful infant eyes that explored the world around him with curiosity and awe. He felt his warm enthusiasm for this tiny new life dissolve into sadness over his uncertain future, as he passed him back to one of the midwives and bade them all farewell.

When he came home and told me of what had happened that evening, I cried for this little one, who was soon to be handed over to others so far away. I sensed a tearing of my heart at the thought of such lonely abandonment of one so young.

We read our own kids some longer stories, and gave them extra hugs and kisses, when we settled them both at bedtime on that particular night.

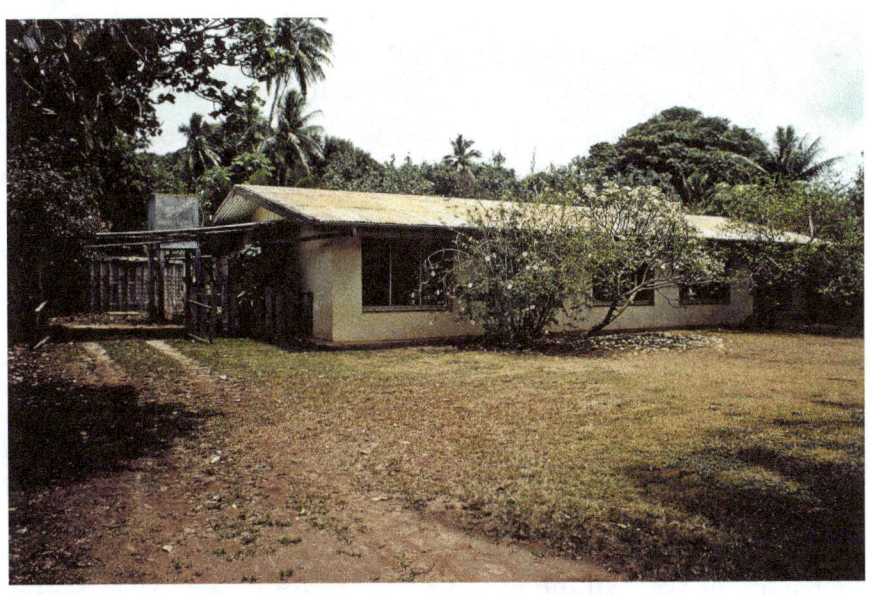

Our house with handmade fences near carport. Note the concrete water tank with metal rungs on the left-hand side of backyard.

17 – Devious Devices

As the middle of our first year on Aitutaki drew near, we received a call from the Minister for Health. He asked if Mike would be willing to return to Raro for two weeks in late June to relieve the country's only anaesthetist, who was going on an overseas holiday.

Mike had given numerous anaesthetics when working in Canberra hospitals prior to our posting, so this role was quite familiar to him. But his former experiences had also made him wary: he had the distinct impression that the Anaesthetics specialty was a curious blend of boredom and terror, but it was the latter that stayed more firmly etched in his memory. Consequently, he was ambivalent about the proposed arrangement.

A week later, the Minister rang back to add that the Department was willing to cover the accommodation expenses for all four of us to stay in a family unit in Raro, since it was similar to Mike's costs alone, and we could pay for our own airfares and meals. This concession made his request more enticing and, after further discussions together, we finally agreed.

Around the same time, an obstetric colleague of ours had sent a letter telling us that he and six others planned to come to the Cooks in late June for two weeks. Denis had been my obstetrician in Canberra, and he and his wife Jan had become good friends since that time.

'They're actually going to be in Raro at the same time as us,' I read to Mike from their letter one lunchtime, 'And surprisingly enough, they're due to fly to Aitutaki on the same date that we'll be returning too. How good is that?'

Mike read over my shoulder: 'Sure is – and it looks like they need us to arrange some accommodation too. Maybe we can check with Father Luke tonight when he and Bonita come over.'

Our friends both had their own news to share that Tuesday evening. Luke knew of a family in his parish who owned a roomy place that they might rent to our friends, and Bonita announced that her parents were also planning to visit her shortly.

'They're going to need a place to stay as well,' she said, 'There's no way that they can fit into my tiny bed-sit.'

I considered this briefly, then suggested: 'If your folks could stay at a guesthouse for a few days, then they could use our house and car while we're in Raro.'

Things seemed to be falling into place for all of us, and we looked forward to meeting each other's acquaintances.

We met Bonita's parents before we flew to Raro in late June. Bob and Ruby were charming folk, but they were rather puzzled by various facets of island life. When they came to our place for a meal soon after their arrival, Bob said: 'Do you know the ceiling fan in our guesthouse just about stops whenever Ruby uses her hair-dryer?'

'Yeah, that kind of thing happens a lot,' Mike said, 'Actually, you should try boiling the kettle at the same time as using a frypan – both of them take about three times as long to heat up.'

In fact, electricity supply was always unreliable on Aitutaki – there were frequent spontaneous blackouts, and at other times erratic surges through the system caused us rare, but disconcerting, electric shocks that were thankfully mostly mild. At certain times of day, the drain on the diesel-generated power maxed out and all our appliances worked at low speed – especially if someone on the system was using building equipment like drills or welders.

We noticed Bob and Ruby becoming more relaxed about island ways during their stay. By the time we returned from Raro, they had learned the names of all the *mokos* (geckos) that lived inside our home, how to drive our manual car on the left-hand side of the road and how to smash cockroaches with any available implements. They had even come to terms with the rats in our ceiling and feral chooks in the garden, like true cross-cultural adventurers.

~

Our lifestyle whilst in Raro differed greatly from the slow pace of life that we experienced on Aitutaki. We relished the opportunity to buy clothes, eat Chinese food and get all kinds of amazing things like sour cream and salad vegetables. As always, the other volunteer families generously offered us lifts, information and meals. But it seemed strange to us that the islanders rode past on their motorbikes without waving. On 'our island' everyone knew us and gave us a cheery greeting, but in Raro we looked just like all the other *papa'a* tourists, so the locals ignored us, just as they would do with any other strangers.

Mike's time at Raro was far from light-hearted, however, especially when he decided to head up to the hospital the day before he was due to start work. He checked over the outdated equipment: the perished and leaky valves, bags, pipes and seals of the Boyle's anaesthetic machine, as well as the complete absence of reliable monitoring or resuscitation equipment, all caused him considerable angst.

His first day on the job was a harrowing one, although it seemed deceptively easy to start with. He checked the surgical list on his arrival at the operating theatre – it looked fairly innocuous, beginning with a haemorrhoidectomy. But as the orderlies wheeled in the first case, Mike was dismayed to note two features of the *papa'a* patient that anaesthetists find especially problematic: a short fat neck and a generous ginger beard. It was difficult to maintain a patient's airway if they were blessed with a chubby neck, and bushy beards allowed gases to leak copiously around face masks. Not a good start.

Taking a few deep breaths and with his usual meticulous care, Mike began to set up the anaesthetic trolley. He had been taught by an obsessive old-school anaesthetist in Canberra to prepare for all contingencies, with endotracheal tubes of three different sizes (the middle-sized one being the diameter of the patient's index finger), two laryngoscopes with spare batteries, and syringes pre-filled with the exact doses of appropriate medications. He felt more confident with the calming effect of these well-rehearsed procedures.

However, his initial attempts to insert a spinal block and ventilate by air-bag were unsuccessful due to the patient's portly habitus, and he felt self-conscious in front of the watching theatre staff. The surgeon and some of the nurses discreetly left for a breather, while Mike set about intubating the patient for a more controlled anaesthetic. This required administering a powerful, fast-acting sedative called Thiopentone, followed by a paralysing agent known as Succinylcholine, then inserting a laryngoscope to guide the endotracheal tube through the patient's vocal cords.

The next step was to seal this tube in position before connecting it to the anaesthetic machine throughout the procedure, since patients given these agents could no longer breathe by themselves.

Mike explained his intentions to the theatre nurse beside him as he injected the Thiopentone and the patient rapidly lost consciousness. He then injected the Succinylcholine into the cannula and total paralysis soon followed. As he inserted the laryngoscope with his left hand to visualise the glistening vocal cords, he reached out for his nurse-assistant to place an endotracheal tube into his right hand, only to realise, after a beat, that the theatre was completely devoid of staff and anaesthetic trolley.

He and the paralysed patient were alone in the room and none of the lifesaving equipment was in sight, let alone within reach.

His horror was raw and visceral.

'I have just killed this man,' coursed through his brain with every pounding adrenaline-charged heartbeat. He called out for the staff to assist him, repeating his appeal with more and more volume and agitation.

'Hey, I need some help here – someone – *anyone... Help!*'

He couldn't leave the patient, as he was trying to extend the *papa'a's* neck and use the air-bag as carefully as possible, despite the troublesome beard. He shouted loudly for the life-saving equipment, his voice rising to frank hysteria by this stage.

'Is there anybody there that can help me or *this man is going to die!*'

After what seemed like weeks, but was probably a few minutes, a startled theatre nurse peered around the door. She was irritated at this interruption to her work, as she thought her tasks at that moment included clearing away the contents of the anaesthetic tray.

'I need that trolley *right now*,' Mike yelped hoarsely.

Finally, the staff and surgeon responded, the half-emptied trolley was retrieved and Mike inserted the long-awaited endotracheal tube. As oxygen flowed into the paralysed man, the blood pressure and well-being of both doctor and patient rapidly improved before any permanent damage was done. But the potential disaster was far too close for comfort...

The remainder of the list was a blur, overshadowed by the possible demise of this man, the crushing weight of responsibility Mike felt, and the shattering of any confidence he'd had in the theatre staff to work in the collaborative way that is so essential to anaesthetists.

After the operation, he went to see the burly red-headed patient as soon as he awoke in recovery and anxiously asked: 'So, how are you feeling, sir?'

'Yeah, I'm ok thanks mate,' the man replied. He seemed to be unaffected by his near-death experience that no one had seen fit to describe to him.

'Just one thing though –' the fellow added with a frown.

Mike held his breath. *Not some symptom of serious neurological deficit, please...*

'I've got a *really* sore bum.'

Mike sighed and nodded slowly: 'Yeah, that's pretty normal after a haemorrhoidectomy.'

Thankfully, this terrifying scenario was not repeated, but it weighed heavily on Mike throughout the remainder of his anaesthetic stint. He found it impossible to relax in theatre for the next fortnight, and re-lived the ordeal over and over again.

Our Canberra visitors overlapped with us during our last five days in Raro. We prepared *eis* with the assistance of the other volunteers and met them at the airport as they alighted from their 5 a.m. flight from Auckland.

'Here they come,' I said to our kids as we saw their tired but excited faces.

Jan smiled with delight as we placed numerous *eis* on each guest. 'We certainly didn't expect to see you here at this time of day.'

'Well, we're so glad you've gone to the trouble of coming, that we wanted to be here to welcome you,' I said.

We joined them in taxis to their motel accommodation and chatted about island life over breakfast. They were keen to hear about our medical experiences thus far, and Mike debriefed about his most recent and vivid traumas, since Denis and Jan were both doctors. They were suitably aghast and sympathetic.

Since we knew something of the highlights of Raro, we suggested various options to our friends for sight-seeing, places to eat and where to see the most authentic island dancing, and we joined them whenever possible over the next few days.

When we returned to Aitutaki, we were on the same plane as our friends, and spent the next nine days recommending activities for them there, as well. They rode hired bikes to see the sights and we joined them for long walks, including up Maunga Pu, the island's highest hill that was only 120 metres above sea-level. From this vantage point, we could see the Pacific Ocean in every direction. This view usually induced a cloying claustrophobia in me, as did circumnavigating the entire Aitutaki land mass in twenty minutes by car. The mainland was only 8kms by 2kms with a narrow arm on the east side – so it was a very small island indeed. I told our friends how I sometimes thought that we could have quietly drowned in rising sea levels and no one beyond Rarotonga would have even noticed for several months at least. They nodded knowingly.

During their visit, a nasty motor vehicle accident occurred when a ten-year-old girl was hit by the school bus. She was unconscious when the ambulance brought her into Outpatients and Mike and Dr Rua assessed her on the operating theatre bed. She had a nasty gash down the side of her head, a deformed arm and gravel rashes down her legs. The two doctors inserted intravenous fluids and X-rayed her head and limbs – discovering that she had fractures to her skull, right arm and right lower leg. They sutured her lacerations and made plaster splints for her damaged limbs, then arranged for her to be transferred to Raro Hospital on the next morning's flight, with Dr Rua to supervise. She eventually made a good recovery, I'm glad to say, although she had a long period of rehab in Raro first.

'Come up to the hospital with us tomorrow morning,' Mike suggested, as we finished a meal of traditional food at a guesthouse with our *papa'a* visitors one evening; 'We think you'll find it an eye-opener.'

When we showed them the facilities and introduced them to the staff, Denis and Jan were surprised to see the simple and outdated conditions under which we worked. Denis was kind enough to see some of our patients who had gynaecological or obstetric problems, and the hospital staff responded to their help with a small *kaikai* lunch and speeches to express their gratitude.

Our friends found it hard to believe that we had no ultrasound machine, and that Mike provided obstetric care without a sonicaid, either in the ante-natal clinic or labour ward. They shook their heads as they saw Mike listen for foetal heartbeats using an old-fashioned wooden horn known as a monaural otoscope – something that Denis had not needed to use for many years by this time.

Wind and rain prevailed for the first half of their visit, but the sun eventually returned. We were fortunate enough to have fine weather for our last *motu* excursion with our friends, when they hired the Akitua Resort catamaran for a full day-trip to One Foot Island. In all, twenty-six *papa'as* came along to share in the scenery, snorkelling, and a Māori *umukai* lunch – it was a great way to enjoy our last day together on the beautiful lagoon.

Once again, the hospital staff augmented our *ei* collection for our friends' airport departure the following day, and we bid them a fond farewell after the special time that we had shared.

A few weeks later, we received a letter from Denis and Jan to thank us for hosting them all, and telling us that we could expect something from them in the near future. It sounded intriguing, but a fortnight went by without any notification from the Post Office that we'd received a parcel. By now, we knew this didn't necessarily mean that there was nothing to collect, as the system for informing residents about postal arrivals was arbitrary, to say the least. So, late one morning, I gathered up the children (now aged three and one) and drove downtown to see what was going on.

When I made my request at the counter, the Post Office staff made various non-committal remarks and went in search of the hoped-for delivery. Reappearing after some time, they confirmed that it had, in fact, arrived. Bringing out the small-suitcase-sized package, I was thrilled to read the sticker that listed the contents as an obstetric sonicaid. Fantastic!

However, taking it away would not be quite so easy…

The staff member gave me an implacable stare. 'But you can't take it now, Mrs Dr Browne. It has to be cleared by the Customs Officer.'

'That's ok, I can hang on till he checks it out,' I said calmly.

There was an uncomfortable pause. 'But he's not here,' she replied with a frown.

'No problem – I'll just wait for him.' I lifted my kids onto the counter where they predictably started to bicker and reach for any available objects of interest.

The clerk withdrew to the rear of the sorting room where the other staff gathered and some anxious murmuring was audible in-between the front-counter squabbles.

Another clerk came forward and said more forcefully: 'It would be best if you come another day. He is very busy today. Try again tomorrow – or maybe next week.'

It was becoming clear that the Customs Officer was AWOL. Perhaps he'd gone fishing or concocting homebrew with the hospital technician – but either way, he was obviously unavailable to do his job.

I gave the clerk a steely stare and reiterated sternly: 'I don't care how busy he is. I'm going to wait here till he gets back.'

I knew enough by now about the glacial pace of public service action in the Cooks to take a firm stand and use any ammunition at my disposal. At this particular moment, that happened to be my children who, I was confident, could soon wear down the resistance of any form of islander bureaucracy.

He returned to the back of the room where further discussion took place and churlish glares were directed towards us.

This time, a female clerk approached the front counter, looking worried. 'Look, we don't know where he is or how long he'll be. It could be a few days maybe...' She trailed off into uncertainty then cast an imploring look in my direction.

'I'll wait for as long as it takes,' I declared impassively and folded my arms across my chest; 'This parcel contains a valuable medical device and I'm not going anywhere without it.'

The kids were becoming rowdier by now as it was getting dangerously close to lunchtime.

She retreated and the staff resumed their intense deliberations, while the sound level at the front desk continued to rise. Finally, another postal clerk came forward and asked: 'Is this equipment important for saving lives?'

I sensed a glimmer of hope and leaned across the counter, replying passionately: 'Yes, it's absolutely *vital* for saving lives. Many babies may *die* if we don't have this machine as soon as possible.'

He withdrew again to communicate this information to his colleagues, who kept darting worried glances back at us. By now, the children were throwing pamphlets onto the floor and shrieking hysterically at each other.

The clerk stepped back at last with a promising look on his face.

Over the intense background noise, he shouted: 'We have decided that you can take the equipment up to the hospital and we'll tell the Customs Officer to check it out there when he gets back to work.'

I yelled back: '*Excellent*, you will save *many* lives!'

Success at last... I smiled broadly and lifted the children down.

With palpable relief, the clerk carried the fragile package out to the car and I thanked him warmly as I passed the kids a rewarding banana each. I drove to the hospital with great excitement to show the gift to Mike and Dr Rua.

We unwrapped the many protective layers of padding and found the sonicaid nestled inside. An enclosed note informed us that, on returning to work after their holiday, Denis had felt so guilty that he owned two sonicaids in his consulting rooms when he knew that we had none, that he had packed up one of his own and posted it over to us. It was an outrageously generous gift and we were thrilled to receive it – such a useful piece of technology for our ante-natal and labour ward patients!

Naturally, we sent a card to the Appels at the earliest opportunity to express our immense gratitude on behalf of the whole Aitutaki community.

Suffice to say, the Customs Officer never turned up at the hospital to check out our 'vital equipment.' So much for the strict standards and thorough inspections of the island's public officials, I reflected later with quiet amusement. It was just as well that I had stood my ground at the Post Office that day and that our offspring, as only children can, had rendered their strategic and uncompromising support.

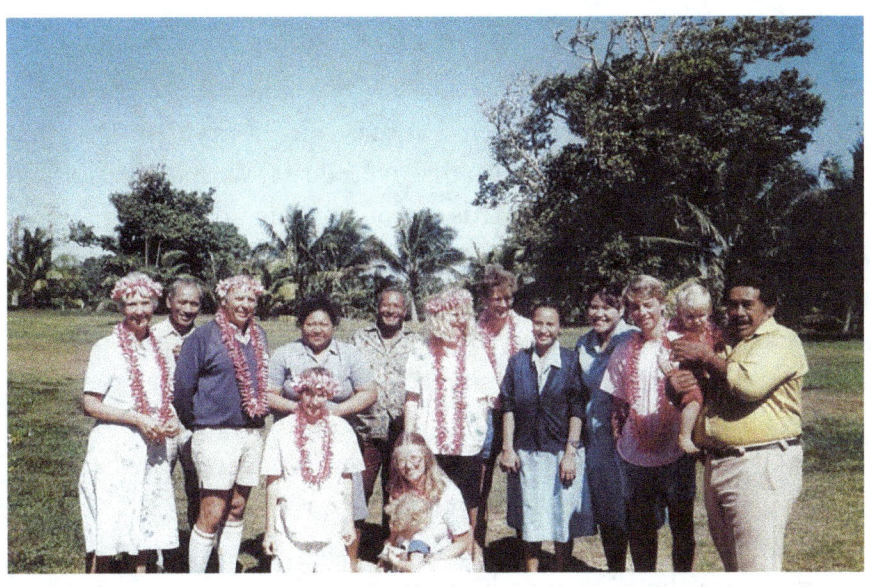

Appels with hospital staff.
L>R Back Row: Jan A, Dr Rua, Denis A, Pua, Rima, KL, Robert A, Tiare, Abi, David A, No'a holding Thomas.
Front Row: ML, Michele, Rhiannon.

18 – Dangers and Delights

We had managed to keep Thomas fenced in during his first year of life, but later on discovered that we had overlooked some further potential hazards for our young adventurer.

One morning, after completing my solitary battle with the wringer washing machine, I emerged from the laundry to make the heart-sinking discovery that our sixteen-month-old son had gone missing. Rhiannon had been immersed in a challenging jigsaw at the time, so she could shed no light on his whereabouts, and Mike was doing his usual Outpatients clinic at the hospital.

It was a desolate and gut-wrenching moment.

But as I searched the house and garden, I discovered Thomas climbing up the nine-foot-high water tank in our backyard and he had now reached the top. Apparently he had found little of interest there, so he'd started to manoeuvre himself downwards, balancing on the rusty metal rungs that encircled the concrete tank. My first instinct was to scream but, realising that this could distract him and cause him to tumble, I shoved a hand to my mouth and breathlessly watched as he made his careful descent.

When he was about six feet from the ground however, he lost his footing and fell. I let out a loud yelp, but was glad to see that he'd landed on some thick springy grass at the base of the tank. Bouncing a little and somewhat winded, he grunted and paused to catch his breath. But not being one to sit still for long, he soon leapt up, thankfully with all four limbs intact, and continued his former explorations.

Feeling limp with relief, I staggered after him and picked him up for a big bear hug. He muttered at me with irritation, indignant that I had interrupted him, and wriggled downwards to resume his exploits. I sighed with a deep sense of gratitude that he was clearly unharmed, and went to the kitchen to make myself that panacea for all life's ills: an urgent and restorative cup of tea.

When Mike returned that afternoon, and I'd told him of what had happened, he set up a ladder against the tank and climbed to the top. There he discovered a large hole about one metre in diameter in the centre of the rusted metal lid. When he descended and reported his find to me, we talked quietly about how close we had come to tragedy that day. The thought that Thomas could have crawled across the top and fallen in, drowning silently while we searched long and fruitlessly for him, filled us both with a sickening sense of horror.

At the first opportunity, Mike went back to the hardware shop and purchased another large pallet. He brought it home, hoisted it up the side of the tank and dragged it over the hole, to deal with yet another hazard for the benefit and longevity of our precious young explorer.

~

Our kids' health issues were a major source of concern for us during our posting. They had several episodes of serious gut and respiratory infections, including bronchiolitis, bronchitis and gastroenteritis. Having two atopic parents, both of our kids had a tendency to tight airways, too; but Rhiannon developed severe wheeze whenever she had upper respiratory infections, and often needed intensive treatment to control her life-threatening asthma.

Thomas also had prolonged coughing after head-colds, but he suffered more from gut infections. He had a few nasty bouts of gastroenteritis and needed intravenous fluids twice during our stay. Due to our concerns about the competence of the hospital staff, we supervised his hydration levels ourselves, by inserting a butterfly cannula into his tiny hand and hooking up the plastic one-litre bags of fluid to a curtain rail at our home.

During one of these episodes, Rhiannon also had the same infection, but not as badly as her brother, so she recovered without needing IV fluids. A few days after his drip began, we knew that our son was on the mend when his sister cried out indignantly: 'Mum, Thomas just hit me!'

It happened to be a good sign on this occasion.

However, these bouts of serious illness were very troubling for Mike and me. It was difficult and far from ideal to be both doctors and parents simultaneously of our own children, especially when they were seriously unwell. But Dr Rua deferred to us on these occasions, not wanting to advise, intervene nor insert a drip into either of our kids, so we had no option but to treat them ourselves, and deal with the conflicting roles that that entailed.

These episodes emphasised our extreme sense of isolation too, reminding us of just how far we were from family and friends, along with medical back-up. At such times, we were thankful for the prayers of others from both near and far, and our faith in One to carry us tenderly through these seasons of loneliness and fear.

~

The Cook Islands were thought to have been discovered and populated during sporadic Polynesian migrations from Samoa and French Polynesia during the seventh and eighth centuries AD. Historians believed that a further mass migration known as 'the great Māori fleet' set out from Rarotonga to other western regions including New Zealand about 1350 AD. The Cooks became a British protectorate in 1888 and became self-governing on 4th August, 1965 (Constitution Day), in free association with New Zealand. Hence, Cook Islanders continued to have automatic New Zealand citizenship.

Constitution Day had morphed into Constitution Week by the time we were on Aitutaki – an annual commemoration of self-governance by the locals that was another excuse for work-avoidance, *kaikais*, drumming and dancing. There was a carnival atmosphere throughout the island, with games similar to those that I remembered from Sunday School picnics of my childhood, including wheelbarrow, egg-and-spoon, three-legged and sack races. Local VIPs were invited to participate in the celebrations and Mike was also asked to speak on behalf of the hospital.

The festivities included a parade made up of floats depicting various aspects of islander life, including our *Tivaevae* group, which had a colourful display of our most recent hand-embroidered bedspreads and cushions. *Tivaevaes* held particular significance for the women who made them, and were highly valued as presents. We still remember the day when a young mother brought one that she had made to our house as a gift. It expressed her sincere thanks to Mike, as his timely intervention with intravenous antibiotics had contributed to her young daughter's recovery from both septic arthritis of the knee and a very serious form of bacterial meningitis. Her daughter had eventually recovered after some months of follow up care, with no long-term complications: it was a cause of much rejoicing for all of us. We were deeply touched by the mama's generosity, and still have this *tivaevae* to remind us of a little life saved and a mother's warm gratitude.

In August 1988, we had a visit from an OSB field officer called Jenny, who stayed with us for several nights. She joined in the commemoration of Constitution Week, as it happened to coincide with her visit. Being in her mid-twenties, she was quite new to her role, but she was a friendly person with an easy manner and we appreciated her good humour and support. We told her about the *tivaevae* gift, along with other highs and lows of our life and work since our arrival on the island. She listened carefully and encouraged us with her feedback. She also spent time with all the volunteers in the Cooks before heading off to other Pacific nations to continue her visits there.

During our second year on the island, she returned for a similar trip, staying this time with our volunteer neighbours next door. On this latter occasion however, she brought the concerning news that one of the other young field officers called Jacqui, who we'd met at the Melbourne briefing, had become very ill during a recent visit to some volunteers in the Solomon Islands.

We were shocked to find out several weeks later that, despite being air-lifted back to Australia for intensive medical treatment, Jacqui had suddenly died. Accurate information was scant, but we eventually heard that she had contracted the dangerous haemorrhagic form of Dengue Fever, a mosquito-borne infection, whilst in the Solomons and it had tragically ended her young life.

Shortly after the end of our posting in late 1989, we heard that there had been a major outbreak of Dengue Fever in the Cook Islands. Seventeen locals died and many others were seriously ill, but eventually recovered. We shared in the anxiety of the local friends who had told us of this grave news. It was distressing to realise that, like them, we and especially our children would have been at risk of this life-threatening disease had we still been on the island at the time, as there were no treatments or vaccinations available for this infection. Like the news about Jacqui's sudden demise, such situations were sobering to reflect on, and posed a deeply personal reality check for all of us.

~

In early 1989, Mike was invited to participate in an unusual overnight prayer vigil organised by a group of islander Christian men, led by the male nurse No'a. Their goal was to visit and pray at various sites called *marae* around the island that had links with Māori traditions from the past, including cannibalism, occult symbols and tribal warfare.

Cannibalism had been a common practice in the Cooks prior to the arrival of the missionaries. Not only was it considered a way of supplementing the mostly protein-deficient diet of the islanders, but it had social and religious connotations too. Our understanding of this practice was that, not only was it important to defeat one's foes, but by eating them, the victors also imbibed their power and wisdom, and thereby weakened or even wiped out the entire enemy population. These beliefs apparently underpinned cannibalism throughout Pacific Polynesian communities.

During their trip from village to village, the small group of men came across a field that contained a huge shallow crater about half the size of a football field. When discussing its history, No'a explained to Mike that approximately one hundred and fifty years earlier, a fierce battle had occurred here between the villagers of Nikaupara and Vaipae. The latter had ultimately won, and the victory was celebrated with an enormous *kaikai*. The crater was where a vast *umu* was built, in which all the inhabitants of Nikaupara were killed, cooked and eaten by the Vaipae tribe. The group spent some time on their intercessions at this place, as they prayed for their ancestors and subsequent generations who had been affected by this horrifying event.

It was a disturbing piece of history, especially since it had occurred relatively recently. We found it unnerving to discover such a gruesome past for this island that now seemed so friendly and peaceful: the disparity made us both thoughtful and thankful in equal measure.

~

Cook Islanders have a great gift for taking all kinds of social events and making them into major celebrations, with food being a quintessential element. These included Naming ceremonies that were observed when infants were about one year of age. Unlike baptisms, these rites were not so much religious as social occasions, like birthday parties, and involved *kaikais*, speeches and singing with typical islander fervour.

Names that were chosen by parents were symbolic or unusual by western standards, even for siblings within a single family. Sometimes, there was a simple reversal of first and second names from one generation to the next: for example, if a father was called Henry Parua, his first son could be called Parua Henry. Family names were interchanged with other relatives' names in the same way, so that four siblings could have four different surnames, even if they all shared the same parents.

Sometimes children were called after the job description of a relative, such as 'Manager,' 'Trainee' or 'Superintendent;' or after their parents' political preferences, for example 'Cook Island Party.' In this case, the Christian name was shortened to 'Party,' which was entirely appropriate for this particular girl! Others named a child after a day of the week on which something significant had occurred for the family, for example: 'Thursday.'

One of the most extraordinary names we ever heard was: *'Mamapapapokino,'* which meant: 'Mum and Dad had a bad night.' I felt truly sorry for the poor girl who had to carry that unfortunate label around with her for the rest of her life!

Another annual festivity was Gospel Day: it celebrated the arrival of missionaries to Aitutaki on 26th October, 1821. Like Constitution Week, there were re-enactments of the historical events, and stalls displaying hand-crafted wooden objects and colourful *tivaevaes*. Drumming, dancing and *kaikais* were highlights as the locals displayed what they did best, with their signature prowess and enthusiasm. It was good to join in with them as they celebrated in their unique and whole-hearted way. When it came to sporting competitions between the villages, we also noticed that Vaipae usually won convincingly and took justifiable pride in its record.

Weddings also ranked highly on the list of important islander celebrations, and we were delighted to receive an invitation from a local couple to attend theirs. Mind you, the invitation was only made verbally to us on the day before the actual event, but that didn't detract from the honour that we felt. The bride was already known to us, as she had attended the hospital antenatal clinic regularly, being now about eight months' pregnant. We didn't know the groom, but he and his family made us welcome when we arrived at the ceremony the following day.

The wedding took place at the Cook Islands Christian Church, and was conducted in Māori with the usual powerful four-part hymn-singing and stirring oratory by the minister. Following this, the bride and groom, who were dressed in western-style wedding outfits augmented by numerous *eis*, seated themselves on a bench seat on the back of a ute that was colourfully decorated with flowers and cushions. The bridal ute drove them from village to village, followed by another truck filled with drummers.

Rhiannon was thrilled when she and Mike were invited onto the second vehicle to join in the celebrations, while I followed in our car with Thomas. Waving regally to the passing villagers and joining in spontaneously with some of the drumming, were both good fun for *papa'a* father and daughter alike.

Locals from each village welcomed the procession, and they came out of their homes with gifts to place at the feet of the bridal couple, usually comprising *tivaevaes*, household furnishings and money. There was much laughter and singing, and many locals ended up at the next destination: the site where the *kaikai* had been set up, with a thatched pandanus roof and flowers decorating the tables. Enormous quantities of food had been prepared, and all the guests wore head or neck *eis* that filled the area with a glorious fragrance.

It was a delightful occasion, and one of several weddings that we were privileged to attend. I was touched that they named their baby daughter 'Michele' when she was born a few weeks later too!

Mid-way through 1988, we received the news that my parents were coming to see us for a fortnight in September, and we eagerly prepared in the weeks leading up to their arrival.

The weekend before their visit, Mike came into the kitchen and held up a couple of wilted green specimens.

'I've only managed to find a few lettuce leaves that've escaped the local vermin,' he said with a sigh, 'I was hoping that we might've had more success with growing veggies during the winter months – but unfortunately, it's as bad as ever.'

I frowned in response. 'Mm, it's very frustrating.'

'Maybe your folks will have some tips for us when they come, since they've had vegetable gardens in so many different places,' he added hopefully.

'Sure,' I agreed, as he placed the leaves in the sink and switched on the kettle. I was rather distracted with another project at the time: I had been given some natural yoghurt culture by one of the *papa'a* teachers, and was learning how to create our own. I read from the recipe, as I mixed up a jar of warm double-strength powdered milk.

'I was thinking of trying to make some coleslaw too, since someone dropped in some cabbages yesterday,' Mike said, as I stirred several spoonfuls of the donated culture into the milk mixture. 'It's a shame we can't get carrots, so it'll have to be just chopped cabbage. Do you think some of your natural yoghurt would be ok as a kind of mayonnaise?'

I looked dubious. 'Worth a try, I guess, but it might taste a bit weird.'

'Yeah, but since we don't have any other kind of dressing, I'll have to make do with an alternative.'

I agreed as I sealed the jar, wrapped it in a towel and placed it in our linen press, according to the written instructions. Apparently, cupboards were considered warm enough for the culture to work in this part of the world, and once it was set, the yoghurt could be refrigerated until the next batch was needed.

'Actually, talking of alternatives,' I said as I came back into the kitchen, 'I thought I'd try to make some sauerkraut with the cabbages too, so that we can have something vaguely crunchy through the summer. It's worth a try anyway, now that we know there are *no* salad veggies here, once the wet season starts.'

Mike nodded as he poured the tea, I picked up the cake-tin and we joined the kids in the living room.

Thomas stared longingly through the louvre windows, hoping to see something large and loud driving past. Since our house was located four hundred metres from the local Public Works depot, he had the joy of watching a steady procession of heavy machinery roaring past our place on most weekdays. They travelled to various projects around the island and threw up clouds of dust in their wake. He had learnt the different sounds made by the engines from memory by now, and was able to announce the name of each one, even before it came into view: 'Fire truck... Big digger... Tractor... Tow truck... Ambliance... Bobcat...' and so on, with remarkable accuracy.

He also relished any chance of clambering over these large machines whenever we came across them randomly parked around the island: they were like playground equipment to our small enthusiast. Of course, they were never roped off, so he could stand on the massive shovels, climb over the tyres or sit in the seats pretending to drive these 'hooge 'normous diggers' as he called them – all sources of immense pleasure to our son. But sadly, no vehicles were visible just then, so he soon gave up and came over for cake instead.

Rhiannon was working on her latest creations: paintings of local scenes and a welcome card for her grandparents.

'Come and see what I've made, Dad,' she said.

'Hey – that's nice. Where would you like to put these ones?'

We were running out of space for her numerous productions – almost every wall was adorned with them, although I had also used some as wrapping paper for her friends' birthday presents, or to cover our dried-milk tins so that they could serve as kitchen canisters too.

'Nana and Pa can take them home for my cousins,' she announced firmly.

'Good. I only hope they've got plenty of room in their suitcases.' Mike grinned and turned to me: 'By the way, what are you thinking of having for dinner to welcome your folks when they arrive?'

'Well, I've had a thought that I could try,' I said, smiling with pleasure at my latest idea: 'What about pizza?'

Everyone looked up in surprise.

'Oh yeah – sure,' Mike snorted, 'And where do you plan to get one of those?'

'Well, I thought that if we called in at the small bakery in Vaipeka, we could buy some uncooked bread dough for the bases. We've got a few tomatoes and onions from Moana, so I could make some pasta sauce, and – believe it or not – we've even got some bacon and cheese in the freezer. Put them all together and we've got –'

'*Pizza*,' shouted Rhiannon.

I smiled at her, as she shared my enthusiasm for this new project. 'I think that all kinds of stuff could work well as toppings – and it gives us a few more meal options when we're desperate for a change.'

Actually, this idea proved to be remarkably successful. Indeed, over the course of the next eighteen months, we discovered that just about anything – even corned beef, *rukau*, *kumara* and spam – was more agreeable when fashioned into pizzas, so it proved to be a delicious and worthwhile experiment.

A short time later, we had the joy of welcoming my parents to the island – they had specially brought suitcases laden with treats to supplement our supplies. We now had our own excuses to have some time off work, eat fish and chips, play card games, as well as showing off the beach, lagoon and other island highlights. The kids showed Bruce and Marguerite how to mash up pawpaws into our yoghurt and sprinkle hand-grated coconut on top as well.

Rhiannon was skilled at conning them into giving her extra attention too: 'You could read me two books this time – that would be faster than just one.' It only made sense to a three-year old, of course.

As part of her role of orienting them to island life, she explained that Thomas was a 'wild crazy boy.' This was demonstrated in numerous ways during their stay, but more especially when he was caught in the act of throwing Mike's mouth organ into the toilet. It didn't sound quite the same again after that brief watery episode.

My parents assisted us in catching and cleaning the local chickens, having been keen poultry owners for many years. During their stay, we were thrilled to snare the best target of all: the alpha-male speckled rooster. This bird had frequently woken us up from 4 a.m. onwards with his maniacal crowing, and we therefore regarded him with a great deal of antipathy. Although he'd proved to be a wary prey, having adroitly avoided our chook trap for months on end, he'd finally succumbed to the beguiling pizza scraps that we placed beneath the screen.

We discovered when we ate him that he'd been the target of another hunter during his adventurous life, when we came across numerous lead pellets in his sinewy body. It seemed that someone else had tried to eliminate him already, probably for the same reason that we had, but clearly they'd resorted to a shotgun instead of a chook trap. However, *we* were the ones who finally succeeded in defeating this wily foe, and thereby enjoyed the inordinately tough, but tasty, rewards for our labours!

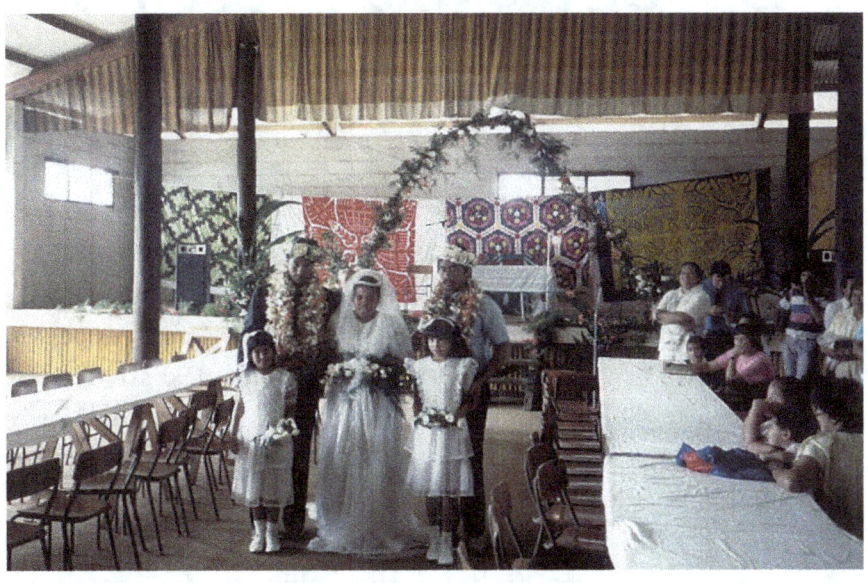

A wedding that we attended.
***Tivaevaes* are being used as background decorations.**

19 – Births and Breeches

During our posting, there were 106 babies born on the island – quite a high birth-rate for a population of only 2,300 people. Thankfully, there was no loss of life of mothers or babies over that period; however, difficult births and especially breeches caused Mike considerable angst at times. In fact, he attributes most of his current grey hair to challenging deliveries in Aitutaki labour ward, so it seems he's still paying the price for these character-building episodes.

A breech is where, instead of being head down (vertex), the buttocks or lower limbs of the baby are the presenting parts. Delivering the lower half of a breech is usually fairly straightforward, but because the head is the largest part of an infant, it can become obstructed in the birth canal, leading to serious problems for both mother and baby. For these reasons, planned caesareans were generally the preferred method of delivering breeches in most countries, both then and now.

Mike diagnosed five breech pregnancies in Aitutaki before labour began, so these mothers were sent to Raro for elective caesareans. But he dreaded discovering a breech in a woman who was already in established labour, as it was too late by that time to get them off the island, and then the problem landed fairly and squarely on him.

~

The insistent revving of the ambulance in our driveway demanded our attention during our lunch on Christmas Day 1988, and we all moaned with dismay at this interruption to yet another family event. As Mike clambered into the cabin, the driver briefly announced: 'Mama having *pepe*.'

As he walked into labour ward, he found a woman who he had never seen before, as she hadn't attended any of the hospital's antenatal clinics.

He waited for a contraction to pass, then introduced himself and said: 'Hello Mama, where have you come from?'

'New Zealand – I arrived in Aitutaki two days ago.'

The midwife passed Mike the antenatal card from an Auckland hospital that carefully documented her visits there and consistently stated that her infant was in a vertex position.

'So Mama Ki, you decided to come back here to have your baby, did you?' he queried with a sigh. He had noticed previously that other Māori women had pursued this same sentimental course of action.

'Yes, it's my birth island, so I wanted to have my baby here too.' She wiped her damp forehead with the back of her hand.

It seemed patently trite at this stage to describe her decision as imprudent – let alone point out that she had deliberately deceived several airlines by lying about how advanced she was in her pregnancy. Mike decided to press on with other lines of enquiry instead.

'Have you had any other *pepes?*'

'Yes, a girl two years ago – no trouble at all.' She gulped from a glass of water in the sultry ward.

'I'm relieved to hear it,' he said, then murmured to himself: 'If you're going to come back to our primitive facilities on a public holiday, the least you can do is to have a straight-forward delivery.'

As he checked her swollen abdomen however, he noticed a neat transverse scar across her lower belly that looked suspicious.

'What happened there?'

'Ah, that's where they cut my first baby out. Her heart kept slowing down, so they did a caesarean, but she was fine.' The mama clearly failed to appreciate any serious implications for her present delivery.

'Right – so it wasn't quite "no trouble at all" then, was it?' Mike muttered, frowning with frustration, but the mama ignored him as she breathed steadily through another contraction.

When it eased, he checked the baby's heart sounds with the recently-arrived sonicaid. We didn't have any transducer gel, but had discovered that coconut oil worked just as well to transmit the sound of the foetal heartbeats. Mike was surprised to note that the infant's heart sounds were loudest in the upper uterus.

'Mm, I'll need to do an internal check,' he said cautiously, 'I've got a feeling that your Kiwi midwives were wrong about your baby's position.'

The mama wiped her face down with a damp cloth, then Mike did a vaginal examination and felt a small scrotum through the opening of her cervix. This tiny presenting part confirmed that, contrary to the Kiwi record, the baby boy was, in fact, in a breech position.

The sum of all these factors: a past emergency caesarean, no previous vaginal deliveries, established labour, no flights available off the island and an undiagnosed breech all combined to cause him a host of horrors. Although he was tempted to have a *papa'a* rant about it all, he knew that it was useless – no one either listened or cared. There was nothing he could do but to settle down, do his best, and to hope and pray that that would be enough.

'Mama Ki, I need to explain the situation to you – your baby is in a breech position and therefore your delivery is going to be much more difficult and dangerous than usual. Also, because you've never had a vaginal delivery before, we'll have to hope that the baby's head doesn't get stuck. I'll need to use some uncomfortable techniques to try to stop that from happening.'

The mama nodded pensively as the unexpected downsides of her decision to return home began to dawn on her.

Then he realised that there was more: 'And by the way, because it's Christmas Day there aren't any flights off the island for two days, so we'll have to pray that it all goes really well.'

The assisting midwives immediately dropped their chins to their chests and began some fervent Māori prayers that lasted for several minutes. Mike was grateful that at least Someone would be helping him out here – Divine Intervention was definitely welcome.

After gathering up some gear from the dispensary, he returned to prepare for her complex delivery. First, he inserted a urinary catheter, as an empty bladder takes up less room in the pelvis than a full one, leaving more space for the foetal head for later on. Next, he gave the mama a spinal block using Heavy Nupicaine between her lower vertebrae, hoping that it would provide good pain relief for the long hours ahead.

He then foraged around in our office for his trusty textbook of practical obstetrics. When he had worked for two months in the New Guinea highlands in 1981, he had found this hands-on manual extremely useful. It was poignantly blood-stained from some of his previous difficult deliveries – an encouraging reminder that, not only had *he* survived some scary obstetrics in the past, but more importantly, so had the mothers and babies.

Mama Ki laboured on for many hours through the night, and Mike regularly checked on both her and her baby between rare snatches of sleep, when he lay down in a spare hospital bed nearby. At about 4 a.m., he did another internal check.

'Mama, you're now fully dilated so you'll need to start pushing soon. I'm going to put in some local anaesthetic and give you an episiotomy to help things along. I'll also need to slow down the delivery of the *pepe's* head so that it doesn't come out too quickly. We'll need to work together on this, huh?'

The exhausted mama nodded and Mike proceeded with an injection and a generous incision of her perineum. It was now time to put the Mauriceau–Smellie–Veit manoeuvre into action. Once the baby's legs were delivered, he inserted his left hand into the mama's vagina and placed one finger into the baby's mouth to pull his neck forward and used his right hand to carefully ease out the head. Thankfully, the mother pushed well, despite all of these intrusive procedures, and the baby boy made his appearance at last.

Nerve-wracking fatigue washed over Mike and the shattered mother wept with relief that her ordeal was finally over. However, the best part of all was the raucous howl from the baby boy that heralded his arrival: it proved to be a thoroughly powerful and triumphant sound!

Part of the strict observance of Christian practices on the island meant that no commercial flights were permitted to or from

Aitutaki on Sundays. Naturally this placed huge pressures on us, if residents had major medical issues between 5.00 p.m. Saturday and 9.00 a.m. Monday. Our job was to keep patients as stable as possible until the next domestic flight, since there were no other means of getting residents off the island, no matter how serious their conditions happened to be. It was truly uncanny how often Mike would be assessing someone with a complicated or life-threatening condition, and simultaneously hear a background roar, as the last plane for the week surged above us, winging its way back to Rarotonga.

That's when he knew he was *really* on his own.

Another sentimental Māori primip (or first-time mother) returned to Aitutaki about her due date with an antenatal card from her New Zealand obstetrician declaring that her baby was also vertex. Saturday afternoon drew her like a magnet to labour ward and the last flight for the week powered overhead as Mike puzzled over the curious position of her unborn babe. His vaginal check confirmed that her infant was breech, but he couldn't find the infant's feet at all.

We had no X-ray facilities at the time, so checking the baby's position radiologically wasn't an option. Between hefty contractions he probed further however and finally realised that the baby boy's legs went directly upwards, with his feet alongside each ear: a very tricky position indeed. An immediate caesarean was the treatment of choice in most places around the world for this presentation – but not here and not now.

A dense cloud of anxiety settled over him as he gloomily anticipated another long and stressful night, reflecting yet again that he had to sort it out without any backup. He inserted a spinal block to relax the young mama and she laboured on for many hours, until she was fully dilated and it was time for Mike to intervene in the delivery.

Once again, his practical textbook of obstetrics assisted, describing techniques to hook a finger around the baby's legs one at a time between contractions, and gently manoeuvre each foot downwards. Mike followed these instructions and, once both feet were in the vagina, he delivered the lower limbs, trunk and shoulders. Slowing down the expulsion of the infant's head with enormous care, he finally eased him out.

Relief and gratitude flooded over him as the infant and his mother howled together at the conclusion of their trial. Afterwards, there was the tedious suturing and cleaning up to be completed, but for now it was all weary smiles, back patting and congratulations around the labour ward.

Although he was exhausted by this time, Mike still needed to give me an extensive debrief of his experiences through a blow by blow account of each detail on his arrival home. Eventually, he was able to unwind enough to fall into a few hours of fitful sleep, replenishing his dwindling energy reserves, before another workday began.

Several days later, he was back in labour ward again – this time with three women in labour simultaneously. The first two births proceeded quite quickly, but the third was a very different story. To his horror, Mike realised that this was his second undiagnosed primiparous breech within a week – although with our continuing lack of X-ray facilities and confusing findings on vaginal examination, he struggled to determine exactly what position the baby occupied.

Thankfully, the teenage mama was only having erratic contractions at that point and, miraculously for a change, there was a seat available on a domestic flight some hours later. Mike arranged for her air-transfer and she was promptly driven to the airport by ambulance and flown to the main island. He found out later that the Raro Hospital X-rays revealed a footling breech, with the right foot and the left knee as the infant's presenting parts. This posed a high risk for mother and baby, so she had an immediate caesarean on her arrival there.

Thankfully, there was another successful outcome, but he was very relieved that this time, others had had to deal with the complex challenges for a change. It saved yet another premature crop of grey hair from popping up on his scalp!

~

The challenging deliveries continued on with erratic persistence…

It happened to be another Saturday afternoon when a further memorable delivery occurred, as one of the young staff members arrived at the hospital, having missed most of her scheduled antenatal checks. She was a teenager in her first pregnancy and was clearly in established labour when Mike arrived to see her. Once again, the final flight for the week was passing overhead when he assessed her, and his internal examination revealed that her baby was also in a breech position.

The dissipating rumble of the plane's engine reminded him that yet again, he was in for a long and lonely night.

To fill in the time, the two senior midwives munched on sandwiches and slurped their tea, as they sat on either side of the young mama's swollen belly, in rapt conversation with one another.

'Do you remember that woman, Mata from Ureia, about five years ago,' Kata began, 'She was in labour for days 'cos the baby was the wrong way round. That one went bad, didn't it? The boy never walked or talked.'

'Yes, I remember that. He still just stays at home all the time…' Abi heaved a sigh.

'And what about the Vaipae woman Pepi, four years ago last

summer? She had a breech too.'

'I was in New Zealand then. What happened to her?' Abi sipped her tea.

'Ah...' Kata gave a long pause to heighten the drama of her story: 'Very sad. The baby died and the mama has never been alright after that.'

'Mm, too bad. There was the one from Amuri village as well – Toru's girl. She was just fifteen – in labour for more than two days.'

'Oh yes – and *that* baby died too.' The midwife shook her head pensively. 'Not good, not good.'

Abi's face brightened with another memory: 'And then there was that mama six years ago – Topi from Vaipeka. She was in labour for *three* days, I think. They flew her to Raro but...'

A depressed shudder followed.

'Yes, that was *sooo* bad. They both died, didn't they?'

More sighs and dismal groans followed.

Mike left for a while to compose himself after this discouraging interchange, and searched in the dispensary for the items he needed for a spinal 'saddle' block. When he returned, he inserted the local anaesthetic solution into the fluid sac that enclosed the girl's spinal cord and prepared for a possible emergency caesarean. Whichever way things went, he reasoned, she'd be better off with her pain well controlled.

Throughout the long night, Mike heard the soft whimpers of the teenager and the mumbled drone of the midwives as they trawled through their recollections, sharing countless stories of obstetric disasters across the mama's contracting belly. He occasionally lay down on one of the empty hospital beds, but sleep eluded him. The strain of knowing that the most difficult part of the delivery still lay ahead weighed heavily on him. His anxiety buzzed insistently like the mosquitoes around his face and, when it became overwhelming, he'd pull on his shoes and return to labour ward for another check on his young patient and her baby.

Hour after hour the mama laboured on, until she began to bear down in the early hours of the morning. With the benefit of a large episiotomy and careful untangling of the infant's legs, Mike gradually drew the baby's body downwards and gently eased out the head. With a lusty cry, the four-kilogram baby girl was born at last and relieved smiles and exclamations bubbled through the ward, engulfing them all.

Afterwards, there was the inevitable episiotomy repair and clean-up to be done. But finally, as he walked down the hill to our home, splattered in blood and chilled by the early morning mist, he felt a rush of elation and gratitude that superseded his exhaustion and flowed through his being. This was not another tragic story to add to the midwives' extensive trove, but a precious little life safely delivered into her island home and blessing the quiet dawn.

20 – Blue Babies and Bluff

I arrived at Outpatients for work one morning to find an unusually large number of patients milling about the hospital for no apparent reason.

'Has there been an outbreak of gastro or something else that I haven't heard about?' I asked one of the nurses, Tua.

She laughed in reply. 'No, it's just Dr Lauf – he's come over from Raro. He always wants to see all the people with diabetes and blood pressure trouble.'

I looked at the growing crowd. 'Ah, well that's quite a lot of folk. But why are all the school kids here as well?'

'He likes to see them too – I don't know why. He's doing a "study" I think, to write down how they're all going.'

'So how long has this "study" been running for?'

Tua seemed uncertain as she considered: 'Maybe seven years now? Anyway, a long time, I think.'

She disappeared into the crowd and I shrugged, thinking that the cardiologist would probably touch base with me later on in the day, to discuss our patients together.

Half-way through my Outpatients' list, I went to get some morning tea and saw Dr Lauf in the staffroom flipping through a pile of patient records. I'd only met him once during our short time in Raro, so I didn't feel that I knew him very well.

'Do you want to talk about some of the patients?' I asked him cautiously.

He frowned at me and snapped: 'No, why would I?'

'Well, we've been treating these people for a while now, so we might be able to share some of their medical information with you.'

'I know what I'm doing with them already.' He spoke in a clipped Germanic accent.

I made myself a sandwich and some tea. 'I understand you're doing a research project of some kind, is that right?'

'Yes, I'm getting population data on diabetes and hypertension in islanders.'

'Right – well let us know if we can help in some way,' I said politely as I took my snack back to Outpatients. I heard a loud snort as I left the room and smiled to myself – it seemed the man had issues of some sort.

A few days later, when Mike came home for lunch, I could see that he was fuming.

'I reviewed a young woman this morning that our Raro consultant saw the other day. I've been keeping an eye on her because her blood pressure's been a bit high.'

'Mm?' I lifted Thomas down from his high-chair and wiped the tray.

'Well Dr Lauf has seen fit to start her on *five* antihypertensives in one go.'

I was astonished with this news. 'Right, well that sounds quite courageous.'

'It sounds like lunacy to me!' Mike could scarcely contain

his pique. 'And what's more, most of those drugs were just sample packs, so as soon as she runs out of them, you-know-who will have to manage with the only brands that we've got in our dispensary here. She's the fourth person I've seen like that so far this week.'

He sighed and I gave him a reassuring smile, for all the good that would do.

'I know what you mean – it's been happening to me too. Unfortunately, the patients get so confused with all these changes, and then we end up just putting them back onto their original treatment after all. It *is* very frustrating.'

I offered to make him a consoling cup of tea.

~

One Wednesday afternoon some months later, when Dr Lauf was visiting the island once again, Mike was checking on some of the in-patients in the ward. One of the nurses found him there and reported: 'A mama and *pepe* have just arrived in Outpatients.'

He followed her out and called them into our clinic room.

'Hello there, what seems to be the problem?' he asked, as he helped the young mother to unwrap her tiny infant on the examination bed.

'My boy Timi was born three weeks ago in Raro. But he came a month early, so he's still very little. I bring him over to see family here, but now he's getting bad cough and looks sick.'

Mike examined the baby and was immediately concerned to see his bluish (cyanosed) lips and hands, and his rapid noisy breathing. As he listened to the infant's gasping chest, he heard a loud heart murmur and crackles of fluid throughout his lungs.

'Did the doctors in Raro say they were worried about Timi before he went home from the hospital?'

'No, they say he got a heart noise but it will get better. But you think he's not good, huh?' She seemed unnerved by Mike's anxious expression.

'Mm, I *am* worried that he's got a problem with his heart,' Mike replied, 'But we've got Dr Lauf here at the moment – he's a specialist for hearts.'

The mother nodded quickly: 'Yes, he saw Timi at Raro before we went home from hospital. He say it's all ok.'

'Ah,' Mike said, thinking of how awkward the situation was becoming; 'Well I think he should check Timi again, before he flies back to Raro this afternoon. I'll see if he's still here.'

Dr Lauf was about to get into an ambulance to go to the airport when Mike spotted him, and asked if he'd come back to see the baby before he left. The cardiologist was irritated that he was being held up, but agreed to review the infant, while Mike found a nurse to ring the airport and ask if they could hold his flight for an extra half-hour. Fortunately, the pilots were quite cooperative about such things, we had discovered.

Examining the baby together, Mike said: 'I'm sure he's got some form of congenital heart disease and it sounds as though he's going into heart failure with fluid in his lungs. In fact, I think he probably needs to be transferred urgently to Raro and maybe even Greenlane in New Zealand. What do you think?'

He was silently willing the specialist to agree with him, and even to offer to take Timi with him back to Raro immediately. He listened hopefully to the other's opinion.

However, Dr Lauf disagreed. 'No, I don't think he's got a heart problem at all. He's just got a chest infection and needs some antibiotics. He'll be better in no time.'

He rolled up his stethoscope and stared at Mike impatiently.

'Oh, ok then.' Mike was surprised at the consultant's summary, but was prepared to defer to his expertise.

'Anyway, I've got to go,' Dr Lauf declared and left to catch his flight without further delay.

Initially, Mike felt relieved with the cardiologist's opinion. This didn't last long however, as Timi's condition rapidly deteriorated, despite the addition of intravenous antibiotics, diuretics and continuous oxygen to the baby's regime. Because of Timi's prematurity, the appropriate quantities of his medications were minute, and the nurses didn't know how to draw them up. So Mike made 'demonstration syringes' and stuck them onto a poster next to the cot to assist in the dosing regimes.

Soon afterwards however, the tiny infant began to have respiratory and cardiac arrests, despite the increased doses of his medications. Mike had to stay with him continuously to manage the recurrent and stressful resuscitations throughout the Friday night.

Returning home for a short shower and change of clothes early on Saturday morning, he poured out his distressing saga to me of the previous night's horrors. I debriefed as calmly and quickly as possible, before he dashed back to the hospital to resume the battle for this little one's life.

Mike arranged the transfer of the now critically ill baby and his mother to Raro on the first domestic flight on Saturday morning. He intubated Timi, packed an oxygen cylinder and resuscitation kit and accompanied him on the transfer to keep his condition as stable as possible. He also asked the pilot to fly at less than 3000 feet to maintain the baby's oxygen levels in the unpressurised cabin. I phoned ahead to ensure that they were met by an ambulance on arrival and taken straight to Raro Hospital.

During the handover at Rarotonga, Mike asked Dr Lauf to assess the baby again. The consultant finally conceded: 'You know, this baby *may* have a problem with his heart.'

Mike was outraged at this reluctant and delayed acknowledgement from the cardiologist, but he managed to contain his exasperation. 'Well, *I* think he needs to go to Greenlane as soon as possible,' he said firmly; 'I've been trying to keep him alive for the past four days, but he needs intensive care if he's going to survive any longer.'

The consultant said nothing as he stared at the infant's heaving chest, while the hospital staff nodded. Mike had a quiet word with the weeping mother before heading off to find transport back to the airport for the flight home. It was a huge relief for him to pass on Timi's care to others after such a stressful ordeal.

It took us some time to discover the final outcome of this situation, as the mother was only visiting family on Aitutaki when her baby became unwell. But we later heard that, by the time he was transferred to New Zealand, it was too late to save him and Timi died several days later. It was a distressing outcome for everyone involved, and Mike took the news especially hard.

~

During another visit to the island by Dr Lauf, Mike had gone to the hospital one afternoon to check on some in-patients when he overheard the sound of a suction pump coming from the operating theatre. He went to investigate this unusual occurrence and was alarmed to see a ten-month-old boy having a grand mal fit on the theatre floor, cyanosed (bluish) and rigid, with intense jerking movements.

Dr Lauf was watching a nurse suctioning the foam around the baby's mouth, Dr Rua sat nearby writing a referral letter to Raro Hospital, while the worried parents stood at the back of the room, aghast with fear. The wild activity of the baby contrasted so starkly with the immobility of everyone else that Mike felt an overwhelming need to act.

'How long's the fit been going on for?' he asked.

'About twenty minutes,' the nurse replied.

'Do you want me to help?' He looked at Dr Rua who nodded eagerly in response, while the cardiologist averted Mike's gaze.

'I need an ampoule of Valium *now*,' Mike said to the nurse, who dropped the suction device and disappeared. He swiftly set up an oxygen cylinder and placed a mask over the baby's face.

'Can you hold this here, please?' he asked, as the nurse returned – she quickly swapped the ampoule for the mask.

Mike drew up the Valium into a syringe, removed the needle, and inserted the dose into the child's rectum. The cyanosed boy gradually relaxed as the Valium kicked in, and his colour improved with the inhaled oxygen. The convulsion had lasted for about thirty minutes by now – enough to cause possible serious brain damage.

Once the baby's tremors had ceased, Mike lifted him onto the theatre bed. He examined him carefully and discovered that he had both a high temperature and a bulging red eardrum. He turned to the distressed parents and asked after the child's name.

'I think Maru's probably had a febrile fit from a middle ear infection,' he explained to them, 'But to be on the safe side, I think we had better do a lumbar puncture to make sure it's not meningitis or something else.'

Dr Rua nodded in agreement and translated for the parents. Then he helped to fold up the baby into a foetal position, so that Mike could insert a needle into his spine to collect some cerebrospinal fluid. While this was sent to the laboratory, Mike carried the infant to the ward and talked through the various possibilities with his anxious parents, and Dr Rua interpreted again.

Once the technician had checked the specimen and reported that it was normal, Mike conferred with his colleague, and they agreed that their provisional diagnosis of febrile convulsion secondary to a middle ear infection was the most likely cause of the baby's fit. They found Dr Lauf in the staffroom and discussed their conclusions with him.

The consultant looked unimpressed. 'Actually, I disagree. I've seen lots of these cases before and I think he's got viral encephalitis and needs intravenous antibiotics for several weeks. He'll probably have permanent brain damage as well.'

He immediately left the room and flew back to Raro later the same day, without any further discussion. Dr Rua shrugged his shoulders, diplomatically discarded his referral letter and left Mike to talk with the parents about how their boy was progressing.

Later that evening, however, Mike felt relieved and vindicated when he checked on Maru and found him looking happy and afebrile after keeping down his oral antibiotics, Paracetamol and a simple meal.

By the following morning, the little chap was crawling along the hospital corridors and giggling at everyone who picked him up. Mike was elated with this outcome that contrasted so starkly with the specialist's grim prognosis – and especially the obvious evidence of Maru's normal brain function. Later that morning, when he informed the parents that their boy was well enough to be discharged home, they shook his hand and Mike joined in with their expressions of relief and gratitude, and the baby's chuckles of delight.

Mike found himself affected by a Raro specialist's decision on a further occasion during our two-year contract.

He was at home one afternoon crumbing some fish for dinner, when there was a knock on the kitchen door. Opening it with his sticky fingers, he found a young man on the doorstep who wanted to discuss a medical issue.

Pata looked embarrassed. 'I'm worried about a lump on one of my balls and I wondered if you could check it for me?'

It was a good thing that the kids and I were still at the *Tivaevae* group, Mike thought as he listened to the story. He finished preparing the fish while he got further details from Pata, and washed his hands at the kitchen sink. Once he had examined the relevant anatomy, both men discussed their concerns about the possibility of a testicular malignancy.

'Well, we haven't got an ultrasound machine on the island,' Mike explained, 'And it's definitely the best way to look at the lump initially, so you'll need to go to Raro Hospital for that.'

Pata considered: 'Sure, if you think so.'

'While you're there, I think you should have an appointment with the surgeon as well, because he might want to do a biopsy to confirm the diagnosis. He might even want to do an orchidectomy – to remove the whole testis – if he's worried that it's malignant.'

Pata nodded as he processed all the implications that such an intervention might entail, while Mike wrote a referral letter to the general surgeon.

Several days after his Raro trip, Pata brought his report up to Outpatients.

Mike read it with interest. 'Ah, the ultrasound showed a solid lump, not just a cyst. So it looks like we were right to be concerned about a malignancy.'

But Pata shook his head with some confusion: 'I know you said that, but the surgeon thought I didn't need to have an operation. He says I just need some medicine – it's here in his letter.'

He passed it to Mike, who read it through carefully. Indeed, the surgeon had described Pata's condition as an infection and had also gone on to write that, apart from a course of antibiotics, no further investigations or follow-up were necessary. The young man stared at him, waiting for Mike's opinion, in view of this unexpected outcome.

Mike searched for a tactful way to state his disagreement with a colleague. 'Mm, this is quite tricky. We can certainly *try* some antibiotics, but frankly, if the lump remains, we have to consider that it could still be a malignancy, unless you have a tissue sample reported as normal by a pathologist.'

'Ok.' Pata nodded as he began to understand the difficulties of the situation.

'Look, obviously the Raro surgeon isn't willing to do a biopsy, let alone an orchidectomy,' Mike said more firmly, 'So we'll have to get someone else involved. Are you planning a trip to New Zealand anytime soon?'

'Well, my wife and I thought we'd go there in about two months' time to visit the family.'

Mike sighed with relief. 'Ok, good. So how about I give you some antibiotics for now and if the lump remains – and I think it will – I'll give you a referral letter to a Kiwi surgeon to check it out for you.'

Pata nodded in agreement as Mike fetched a few antibiotic kits and wrote a referral letter for a New Zealander surgeon.

We heard no more about the outcome until four months later, when we received a letter at the hospital from a Kiwi specialist that read: 'Pata is making good progress after his surgery and radiotherapy for testicular cancer...'

Mike was filled with a powerful sense of outrage that, once

again, he had been thwarted by a Raro doctor and an unnecessary hold-up in treatment had occurred. He was also worried that this delay could have had serious consequences for Pata's response to his cancer treatment.

However, I'm glad to report that since that time, we have heard that Pata continued to do well and he appears to have made a full recovery, despite (rather than because of) his Cook Islands' specialist involvement.

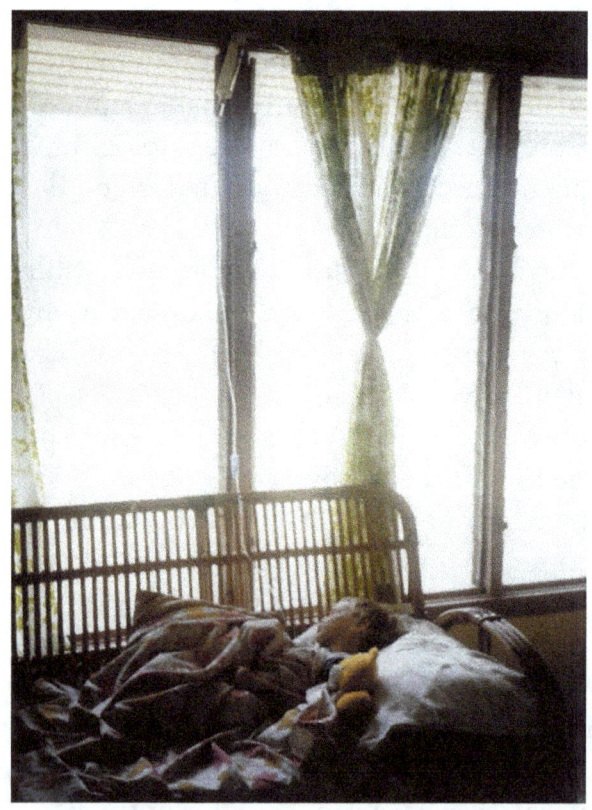

Thomas very ill with gastroenteritis on a drip attached to a curtain rail at our home.

21 – Communication

During our time on Aitutaki, the only electronic means of contacting the outside world was via radio telephone. This rather archaic mode of telecommunications required a telephonist to use a manual switchboard to connect callers from across the Cooks, as well as across the globe.

As usual, we received no explanations about how these telephones worked, so our early calls home to relatives were hit-and-miss affairs, consisting of long pauses on either end, then both sides talking at once. Eventually, we discovered that the telephonist was waiting to hear the word 'over' to indicate when each caller had finished their part of the conversation, so that she could switch the other one through. Once we'd got the hang of it, and explained the magic word to our family members, we generally enjoyed successful calls in both directions.

However, it was rather off-putting knowing that the entire conversation was being overheard by a third party, so this tended to dampen our spontaneity about sharing personal information. The calls were expensive too, so we didn't make them very often, and there was only one channel for phone calls off the island, so they needed to be booked ahead of time. The small-town nature of the phone system indicated the priorities of the various facilities on the island, with the hospital phone number being '2', and our home phone number being '151'. At least it was easy for us to remember our contact details.

The radio phone system for inter-island or international calls was often disrupted by tropical storms. This caused frustrations if we needed to arrange the transfer of patients to Raro Hospital, to ensure that they would be met on arrival and transported efficiently for further care. Sometimes during bad weather, we could only hope that they'd been collected without incident, as we were unable to confirm the outcome either way.

The telephonist, a faceless stranger on the line, was highly skilled at locating local residents – presumably because someone else on the line knew where they were. Likewise, if someone was trying to find us, she seemed to have an uncanny ability to track us down: it felt like an unnerving kind of electronic stalking.

For this reason, we greatly appreciated having occasional overnight stays on Akaiami (the *motu* with a furnished house on it), since it was impervious to hospital demands or telephone queries. At last, we could finally escape the kitchen door consultations and the revving ambulance that summoned us around the clock. It was such a relief to be left alone, at least for these short windows of time.

~

When Rhiannon was about three and a half, she announced that she wanted to start going to Preschool. This activity was conducted on the same campus as both the Primary and High Schools, just across the road from our front driveway. She had heard about it from her little friend next door who had started attending with Rhiannon, but later withdrew. This meant that our daughter became the sole *papa'a* child attending Preschool, and she remained very conspicuous in the crowd of youngsters due to her profusion of tight blonde curls.

Being a stickler for doing things properly, she often insisted on catching the school bus along with many of the other kids. The fact that it was only a two-minute walk from our home to the Preschool building was beside the point for her, so Thomas and I sometimes accompanied her on the bus for a welcome change of scene. This vehicle was aged and battered, and all the seats, although broken and useless, had still been retained on the bus. Consequently, we would have to stand in the aisle, or in front of the damaged seats, or attempt to perch on the residual metal bars. Similarly, the cracked windows were jammed into a half-opened position, so it was often a stifling ride, especially on hot sticky days.

The bus collected us at our driveway, and lurched its way around the island, throwing up clouds of white dust from the crushed coral surface, heaving and straining with each crunching gear-change. We smiled and waved at locals along the way for about forty minutes before arriving back to exactly where we'd started. After alighting in front of our house, we walked along the school driveway and lined up with the other kids in preparation for the morning assembly.

Teachers blew a conch shell to announce the class times, students stood in the open air to sing hymns and traditional songs, and staff made various prayers and speeches. The preschoolers were then herded off to their two large classrooms, where their two teachers supervised about sixty children who ranged in age from three to five years.

Preschool was conducted almost entirely in Cook Island

Māori with a good deal of rote learning and chanting. There were no tables, chairs, paper, pencils, story books, paints, toys or other supplies that would be considered essential in western educational facilities. The only means of writing or drawing was by using chalk on small blackboards that were fixed to the classroom walls.

The Preschool teachers took turns in carrying a narrow rod about five feet long. Mike and I thought at first that it was used to coax the students in various directions when the kids were lining up, a little like herding sheep. But we later saw that it was being used to call the children to attention, when it was whacked against a part of the building with a startling snap. At least it didn't appear to be used on the children themselves, or we would have removed Rhiannon from Preschool immediately.

It was fun to see the kids putting on their occasional performances for the parents, as they recited rhymes, numbers and similar lists. While an adult strummed a *cocophone* or ukulele, they sang songs and did the actions in a somewhat regimental fashion, under the watchful eyes of their teachers.

Somehow, Rhiannon managed to flourish in this unlikely environment and rapidly became fluent in Māori. In fact, she absorbed it so well that she would sometimes come out with quirky remarks like: 'Hey Mum, what's the Māori word for *kaikai?*'

One day, I found her writing down the English names for the days of the week, in her usual phonetic style. I asked her what she was doing, and she explained: 'I'm writing out the *papa'a* words for my teacher, so she can learn the English names too.'

It was kind of her to share her language skills with her teachers in such an egalitarian way, I thought.

In November 1988, we were visited by our two old friends Mark and Karl, who we had known since our student days. Mark had gone through high school then the University of New South Wales (UNSW) medical course with Mike, while I had done the same course in the year ahead of them. We had met Karl when we were all together at Goldstein, a UNSW residential college, in the 1970's.

Mike took a few days of annual leave during our friends' visit: it was a good chance for him to learn to scuba dive, and doing so together with his old mates made it even more fun.

The kids and I waved to the three guys as they set off on the morning of the third and final day of their training, as they cycled down the road to Ned's place. The scuba course was accredited by NAUI and included lectures and examinations on Boyle's Law (volume is inversely proportional to pressure) and other aspects of underwater physics. They had gone on several trial dips inside the lagoon on the first day to get used to the equipment, before progressing on to more serious dives outside the reef on days two and three.

Ned cautioned them when he saw how pumped they were to explore the ocean depths at first-hand: 'Now you need to take things carefully, lads.'

'Yeah, well I tend to get severe pain in my frontal sinuses when I get to about thirty feet,' Mark replied, 'So that slows me down a bit.'

'Pah,' exclaimed Karl, 'This is child's play!'

He rolled backwards off Ned's boat, swooping up and down reef canyons and narrowly missing the sharp edges of coral crests as he powered along.

'Do you have some kind of death wish, mate?' Ned muttered

when Karl reappeared at the side of the boat twenty minutes later, 'I seriously need to warn you that your approach to diving puts you at grave – and I mean, *grave* – risk of either the bends or fatal pulmonary barotrauma.'

Karl gave a long slow smile and nodded calmly. 'Yeah, I should pull my head in.'

'Yeah, you should,' Ned agreed as he pulled on his mask and descended back into the water.

The other two took a more measured approach, exploring the drop-off with their instructor who pointed out some of the remarkable architecture as the reef cascaded downwards into the indigo dimness beyond the sunlight. Once Mike had stopped focusing on his breathing and the panicky dread of equipment failure, he was able to relax into the clear warm water, overwhelmed with the spectacle of the myriad life-forms on display. Brilliant flashes of fish darted continuously around them, in huge clusters that flitted backwards and forwards in effervescent clouds of colour. It was a truly remarkable sight.

They returned to the boat eventually and the four men sat quietly on the trip back through the reef passage to port, humbled by the experience that was beyond words and reflecting quietly to themselves. Ned signed off their course requirements, they settled their accounts and shook hands.

'I'm glad you all survived anyway,' he said, looking pointedly at Karl; 'And I hope your sinuses recover,' he added, laughing at Mark, 'They've certainly had a good wash-out anyway, huh?'

Mark nodded and winced, and Mike sympathised with his mate's headache and facial pain.

'I hope I can do some more dives with you in future,' Mike said.

'Actually, that would be good for me as well,' Ned agreed, 'I'll get in touch about some ideas I've got for an arrangement that could suit both of us.'

Mike nodded keenly and they arranged a time to discuss it further.

Meanwhile, Mark had kept a travelogue of their island holiday that included a description of the scuba course, their many long treks and bike rides around the island, and an overnight *motu* excursion hosted by Grant, 'the *papa'a* Māori', who continued to indoctrinate them in his tried-and-true techniques for catching fish and local women.

During their stay, our friends had also noticed the numerous funny miscommunications that occurred between *papa'as* and Māori, even islanders who had quite good English. I've borrowed from Mark's verbatim record of a phone conversation that happened during their visit as it demonstrated some of these amusing interactions:

Mike: Hello Papa Tarua – it's Dr Browne here. I have two friends over from Australia who want to have some good island food, and I've told them that you have the best. Can we book to have dinner at your place tomorrow night?

Papa Tarua: What do you want?

Mike: To have dinner at your place – tomorrow night.

Papa Tarua: You mean to stay here?

Mike: No, just to have dinner.

Papa Tarua: What time?

Mike: We'd like to eat early because of the children, around six o'clock. Is that alright?

Papa Tarua: (Pause ...) You mean in the afternoon?

Mike: Yes. But if that's too early, we could make it seven. We'd just like to eat fairly early because of the children.

Papa Tarua: So you want to eat at the Rapae Hotel?

Mike: No, we don't want to eat at the Rapae. We want to eat at your guest house tomorrow at 6 p.m. if that's OK.

Papa Tarua: Who is this?

Mike: It's Dr Browne. Can we eat at your place at 6 p.m. tomorrow?

Papa Tarua: Oh – how many coming?

Mike: Our friend Bonita is coming too, so there'll be seven of us.

Papa Tarua: You want to come at seven o'clock?

Mike: No – there are *seven* of us coming. We want to eat at *six* o'clock at your place.

Papa Tarua: OK. We'll see you next week...

Mike: No, we don't want to come next week, we want to come tomorrow.

Papa Tarua: What's your name?

And so it went on... and on... and on...

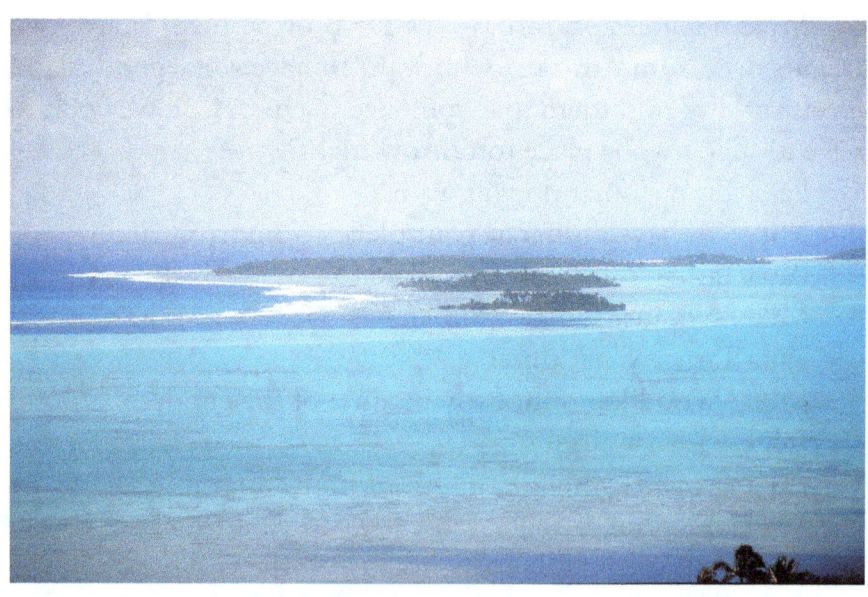

Aerial view of Aitutaki motus and the lagoon.

22 - Solution B

The only form of medical imaging that we had on Aitutaki was a Korean War vintage American Field Army X-ray machine, the kind seen on the old TV program called M*A*S*H. It was designed for use in mobile military tents and hospitals in the 1950's. Accompanying this archaic device was a mouldy set of instructions describing the numerous dials and settings on the machine, to outline the intensity in Kilovolts and exposure time in seconds that was required to image various body parts. For example, an abdominal X-ray required us to hold down the exposure knob for thirteen seconds, which seemed an inordinately long time to us, and no doubt delivered a massive radiation dose to our unfortunate patients.

Whenever he used the machine, and despite wearing the only hefty lead apron that we had available, Mike always felt a strange tingling sensation in his scrotum – no doubt as his testicles recoiled in a desperate but futile attempt at self-preservation.

Mike had to hand-develop the X-rays that were taken in two large sinks in the hospital's darkroom that was lit with a single dim red bulb. He removed the exposed acetate films from their lightproof cases in the darkroom, and attached them with bulldog clips to metal frames that he then immersed into a mixture of two developing solutions. This concoction was made up of a large blue bottle of Solution A to which a one litre orange bottle of Solution B was added, and the two were mixed together in one of the deep concrete sinks with a wooden spoon. After plunging the films into this developing mixture, he put them into a 'fixing' solution in the second sink and then hung them up to dry.

The whole process took about thirty minutes and he found it quite satisfying, being very much like the process he'd used to develop his own black and white photographs at school when he was a nerdy teenager. With our usual turnover of patients needing X-rays, the developing solutions needed to be replaced about once a month. Of course, we had to draw our own conclusions from what we produced, but mostly the images that came into view from those concrete sinks were quite reasonable.

However, about nine months after our arrival on the island, we ran out of Solution B.

This brought our hand-developing to an abrupt halt and rendered our X-ray machine completely useless. We couldn't simply send the undeveloped films over to the main island, as Raro didn't have this system of developing their films, being blessed as they were with a more modern X-ray machine. Consequently, we proceeded to send one order after another for the Raro Dispensary to send through the replacement chemicals that we needed. But once again, we received the same response as our requests for many other supplies: our pleas were ignored, no matter who we contacted on Rarotonga.

The only choice we had, if we felt a patient really needed X-rays, was to send them at government expense on return domestic flights to Raro Hospital to have their imaging done there. This system was a costly exercise in a country with a very limited health budget and an economy that was always in deficit. Therefore, we tried to minimise the number of patients we transferred. If someone had a straight-forward fracture, we'd simply set it with a plaster cast and not bother with X-rays at all, to avoid the unnecessary travel costs involved. In fact, as with the lack of many other resources, we soon learnt to rely more on our clinical judgment than imaging or pathology tests.

It was a trying situation, however, and became even more frustrating as time went by, as it should have been quite simple to sort out. No one could explain to us whether or not there was a global shortage of Solution B, or if it was simply the same old communication issue that we endured with our requests for other medical supplies. Whatever the reason, the situation remained as baffling and unresolved as ever.

Some months after the Solution B crisis began, there was a change of government in the Cook Islands, and a group of newly elected politicians visited Aitutaki shortly after the election results were announced. They expressed support for various projects that they had apparently promised during their campaign. We often found it challenging that, despite the rhetoric of increasing resources for local people, there seemed to be an astonishing lack of genuine change, regardless of who was in power. For example, the public school continued to have inadequate toilet facilities or school supplies, and teachers who had left were often not replaced, causing major problems with under-staffing. Yet politicians came and went with no apparent improvements at all. Perhaps it was not so surprising, as we knew these kinds of scenarios were common in many bureaucracies around the world – including our own back in Australia.

The new Director General of Health, who had done his

medical training in New Zealand, was part of the visiting entourage to the island, along with various public service officials. They sat with Dr Rua and us to discuss a range of matters related to the running of the hospital, including nursing shortages, rosters and internal audits – none of which were issues we felt particularly passionate about.

However, we took the opportunity to discuss the fact that the medical supplies we ordered were so consistently delayed or inappropriate, and then gave special emphasis to the urgent need for Solution B. We pointed out that flying patients to Raro for imaging was an enormous drain on health expenditure that could be better spent in other ways. The politicians nodded as they clarified exactly what we had requested, and emphatically pledged to deal with these matters as soon as possible.

Several months later, when the Solution B remained as elusive as ever, we had another opportunity to raise our concerns. We had been invited to an enormous *kaikai* on the island to celebrate the 80th birthday of the mother of the Director General of Health. While we were at the function, we found the Director and took the opportunity to corner him about the unresolved matter of the Solution B supplies. The politician cheerfully confirmed that he would give it his immediate personal attention on his return to Raro, as soon as the extravagant celebrations were over.

However, we had lived in the Cooks for long enough by now to regard these promises with a fair degree of scepticism, which was just as well, as we heard nothing more for many months. We continued to request the developing chemicals through the usual channels, and zero response followed with monotonous regularity. Our radiology machine lay idle and we grudgingly signed the vouchers to authorise selected patients to travel by commercial flights to Raro whenever we thought they really needed X-rays.

Finally, late in 1989, we received a telegram from the Minister for Health saying that they would be responding to our concerns regarding radiology services on the island in the near future. We allowed ourselves a tiny whiff of optimism, surely not unreasonably so after such a long wait…

Several days later, there was an excited buzz among the hospital staff, who had heard that a delivery had arrived at the port with the latest supply ship. They urged us to go down to the dock to investigate. We hastened there and found a large wooden crate on the harbour-side addressed to the hospital. With the assistance of some enthusiastic locals, we managed to prise open the timber pallets that enclosed the bulky contents. A thrilling shout went up from the islanders when they discovered that the crate contained a slightly newer version of our current outdated X-ray machine, wrapped in plastic layers and sent from some anonymous overseas donor.

'Who on earth still owns a functioning Korean War X-ray machine in 1989?' I asked, unable to disguise the bitterness in my voice, as we stared at the device.

'And why exactly do they think that we'd want *another* one?' Mike said through gritted teeth, feeling just as incensed as me.

After unwrapping the delivery sufficiently to confirm that nothing else was included in the crate, we left it at the docks, overwhelmed with frustration and despondency. The hospital staff, who went on to manoeuvre the heavy arrival onto the ambulance, couldn't understand our profound disappointment at the latest arrival. Surely this machine was just what we wanted, wasn't it?

When we left the island some months later, the 'new' X-ray machine, still enclosed in its wooden planks and plastic coverings, sat in the radiology room alongside the 'old' one. Each was as neglected and useless as the other. After all, despite the promises from the various politicians involved to address the hospital's radiology needs, the crate lacked the one thing that we had continued to request for so long:

There was still no Solution B.

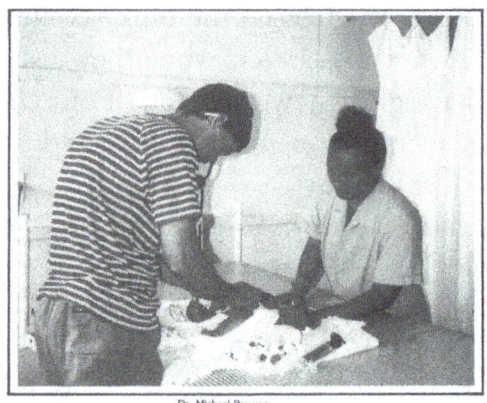

Front cover of OSB's 1987-88 Report, featuring Mike with local baby and nurse at Aitutaki Hospital. Used with the kind permission of Molly Garcia-Underwood, OSB Board and Executive Assistant by email on 9/12/2019.

23 – Christmas and Curious Conditions

During December 1988, there were numerous comings and goings on Aitutaki. Dr Rua had a six-week trip to New Zealand to visit his sick wife, which left us in charge of round-the-clock medical care on the island once again. Our neighbours next door returned to Australia for the school holidays, and their empty house was occupied for a month by the other volunteer family from Mauke whom we had met at our briefings earlier in the year. They were expecting the birth of their third child in January '89. Hearing tales of life on their island made us feel that ours was a bustling metropolis with fantastic access to food and entertainment. These things are always relative, I guess.

Our Mauke friends told us that their island was surrounded by steep cliffs and wild surf, so they could rarely find a beach that was safe to swim in, their only mode of transport was by bicycle, there were few fluent English-speakers on the island,

and they only had electricity for eight hours each day. Mauke shops were usually poorly stocked, so the family seemed to live predominantly on a diet of *kumara*, rice and Weetbix. As a result, they thoroughly enjoyed the range of food, shops and delightful beaches available on Aitutaki. It was fortuitous too that mangoes were in season at the time of their visit and our huge avocado tree dropped six or seven enormous fruits each day. It was good to have others with whom to share such a profusion of tropical delights at this time. We loved having their company, and passed on our baby backpack to them, in order for them to transport their new arrival around Mauke during the year ahead.

We heard some weeks later that, after returning home, the wife gave birth to a daughter on the kitchen floor, as things had progressed rather more quickly than they were expecting. Thankfully, both mother and baby recovered well and had an uneventful post-natal experience, despite the unusual delivery suite!

We felt so conscious of their challenging living conditions that we arranged to send boxes of groceries to them from time to time. On one very thrilling occasion, an entrepreneurial shop owner arranged to have apples flown from New Zealand to Aitutaki, the first that we had seen since our arrival there. They cost three dollars each, so we cut them into quarters and had one segment each, to make them last for as long as possible. It felt like a lifetime since we'd last had something crunchy to eat and we relished every mouthful.

We bought extra apples from the local shop and air-freighted them along with other foods to our Mauke friends, anticipating their excited grins when they opened the cardboard boxes and discovered the delicious contents inside.

Christmas was a very low-key season on Aitutaki. In fact, you could have been forgiven for not even realising it was approaching at all, as there were no decorations, presents, wrapping paper or special foods visible anywhere on the island. We attended a service at the Cook Islands Christian Church on Christmas Eve, at which the locals sang various old hymns as well as six or seven English carols. While the traditional songs were enjoyable, singing with Māori folk about snowy scenes seemed quite incongruous in our sultry summer heat.

Our friends Bonita and Father Luke joined us at the church service, while a neighbour minded our kids. At the inevitable *kaikai* that followed, there were some real *papa'a* cakes for a change in addition to the usual fare, so we grabbed a few slices and surreptitiously escaped home, before the inevitable round of long and tortuous speeches began.

In October, Mike's parents had sea-mailed two large boxes to us on the same day, hoping that they would arrive by mid-December: one contained food and the other one presents. The one containing Christmas food arrived on time and was a great addition to our yuletide festivities. But the second box was unaccountably delayed and turned up in February '89. We were becoming more like the locals by this time, in that it took us little excuse to have another celebration: the belated arrival of the box of presents enabled us to enjoy a second round of low-key revelries. Our kids decided that we should have two Christmases every year and we were inclined to agree with them.

We had recently heard from someone on the island that their parents had celebrated Christmas Day with their relatives in Australia, then flew to the Cooks the following day and had a second Christmas Day with other family members there. It was only possible because of the time zone changes that both days were dated 25th December – but it sounded like a really good way of doubling the fun!

At 8 a.m. on Christmas morning there was a knock at the door, and nineteen-month-old Thomas rushed into the kitchen. He couldn't reach the handle yet, so he simply mimicked the knocking from his side until Bonita pushed the door open.

'Happy Christmas, young man,' she said as she came in, carrying some attractive parcels in her arms.

'You're just in time to open presents,' Rhiannon called from the lounge-room, where our own small pile sat around a casuarina pine tree in a bucket, decorated with simple trimmings that she had painted herself. Since she was now three-and-a-half, she had a keen sense of making the most of every occasion. Mike and I welcomed our guest with mugs of steaming tea and a pile of toast, and the parcels were soon exchanged and opened by everyone.

'What's that present over there?' Rhiannon asked, pointing to a white plastic bag with a small hole cut from one corner and an intriguing portion of black stitching peeping out.

'Why don't you open it and find out?' Bonita replied with a grin.

The kids tore off the wrappings to find a large white Santa bear, replete with a red and green knitted scarf. The fascinating opening had been positioned directly in front of his round black nose.

'He still needed to breathe,' Bonita explained to the kids, 'So I had to make a little hole for him. By the way, his name is Chris – short for Christmas. Someone gave him to me last year, but I thought you guys might be able to give him a new home.'

The kids were delighted and the bear was immediately taken for a ride in the back tray of their indoor trike.

'He's definitely too big for me to take back on my flight,' Bonita added as we watched them playing together.

I felt an ache of sadness at this reminder of our good friend's imminent departure. She had played such a treasured role in our lives since our arrival that it was hard to imagine island life without her.

'Oh, we're going to miss you so much,' I said gloomily.

But Bonita declined to get emotional about her plans. 'Yeah, yeah, yeah. How about we start getting things ready for lunch? What's on the menu, by the way?'

'Well, we were given a hind quarter of pork recently – and we've been saving some spuds for the past few months – so they should go well together,' Mike said.

'No one's been game to eat them before today, or there'd have been *serious* consequences,' I said, then added, 'Mike's folks have even sent us some apple sauce in their food parcel – it was really thoughtful of them.'

I felt quite homesick that day and gave a sad sigh as I imagined our families back home getting ready for their own celebrations.

We headed to the kitchen to start peeling *kumara* and our precious potatoes and putting the pork in the oven. Mac and Ena had sent over a tinned plum pudding and a carton of long-life custard – they were perfect for dessert – while my parents had brought over Christmas crackers and chocolate money on their September trip. The 'money' was a family favourite and despite being past its best, having melted in transit and storage at various stages, chocolate was still chocolate and therefore always highly prized.

Just as our meal drew to a close, the familiar throaty revving of the ambulance sounded from the driveway.

'Oh no, not *today* – it's not fair that Dad has to go to work now,' said Rhiannon with uncharacteristic ire. Pointing to her neck, she said with a look of intense outrage: 'I've had it up to *here* with this place.'

Mike commiserated with her. 'Sorry sweetheart, I wish I didn't have to go either, but someone must need my help.'

He shrugged and gave the kids a big hug before heading out the door. The demands of our working life were much more frequent than usual in Dr Rua's absence and they clearly took their toll on all of us.

A few days later, there was a festival that proceeded from one village to another, with female dancers in matching home-made outfits performing intricate steps along the middle of the road. They were followed by drummers aboard a truck who kept the dancers in time with their vigorous beat. Bonita had joined one of these groups and practised with them twice weekly for six months to learn the complex steps with the other women. She performed admirably and the islanders were delighted to have a *papa'a* join in their display, while we cheered them all on from the roadside. Thomas did his own version of the dances on the footpath too, and his efforts were greeted with appreciative merriment by the good-humoured locals.

Early in January, we bade farewell to Bonita, who had completed her two-year posting of High School Maths teaching on the island. She was going on a trip to Australia and New Zealand prior to returning to her home in Michigan, USA. She was exemplary in her self-control and organisation, but we were very teary when driving her to the airport for the last time, draped in *eis*, knowing that we would sorely miss her genial company, good humour and warm friendship.

I am glad to say that we have kept in touch over the years and even saw her again in the USA in 2017 after almost three decades apart.

In late 1988, our workload markedly increased for no apparent reason. Throughout the year, the record system indicated that approximately 650 patients each month had attended the hospital as either outpatients or in-patients. But during December, when Dr Rua was mostly away, this had increased to 1014, including 54 procedures, and naturally these statistics didn't include the numerous kitchen consultations either. The complexity of cases escalated too, and we often felt overwhelmed and weary as we faced these challenges around the clock and by ourselves for many weeks at a time.

We saw several young people with Rheumatic Heart Disease: a condition that was much more common in Māori than *papa'as*, just as it also tends to occur more frequently in other indigenous populations around the world. One of these cases was a seven-year-old boy, who had developed a serious complication known as endocarditis – a bacterial infection of his already damaged heart valves. This disease required long courses of high dose intravenous antibiotics to bring it under control. Because our supplies were critically low yet again at that time, he needed to be transferred to Raro to receive the full course of treatment. Also, since the small inter-island planes were unpressurised, it wasn't safe for him to be flown at the usual elevation of 9000 feet. Mike asked the pilot if he could fly below 3000 feet, as he'd had to do on several previous occasions, and the pilot kindly agreed. Mike accompanied the boy to stabilise him during the transfer and he made a good recovery after six weeks of treatment at Raro Hospital.

Another run of challenging patients included multiple obstetric deliveries, various fractures, a teenager with pneumonia, another with acute appendicitis (whom we stabilised with IV antibiotics and transferred to Raro), several children with animal bites and burns, various locals with boils and abscesses that needed to be drained, and a cricketer who found out the hard way that he needed to wear a box over his genitals when batting in future!

We often saw local subsistence fishermen with injuries related to their work as well. One man had been pulling in nets without protective gloves when his companion had accidentally turned on the engine of their fishing boat. The net became tangled in the motor and rapidly trapped the fisherman's hand, resulting in a degloving injury to several of his fingers. This meant that the flesh of these fingers was peeled off down to the underlying bones. Because of the serious damage to tendons, nerves and blood vessels that occurred, he was at risk of irreversible dysfunction. Mike gave him pain relief, injected antibiotics and wet dressings before transferring him to Raro on the next day's flight for surgical repairs.

Another local man had a deep laceration from an angle grinder – more tedious hours of suturing were required to pull his tattered tissues together again. On a further occasion, an islander fisherman had injured his hand and was brought to the hospital by his friends. While pulling in a large catch of fish, a stingray in the net had lashed out with its tail, perforating his palm and going straight through to the back of his hand. Although it must have been excruciating, the Māori responded with characteristic stoicism. Mike used a brachial nerve block to anaesthetise his whole arm and surgically removed the complete triangular barb and attached tail. He added antibiotics and tetanus shots for extra defence against possible infection, while the fishermen exchanged tales with each other to entertain their friend.

There seemed to be no shortage of interesting and challenging cases – and although we often felt weary from the unremitting workload, we were continually impressed by the resilience and good humour of the islanders we treated. It helped to compensate for the interrupted meals, diminished family time, and inevitable lack of sleep.

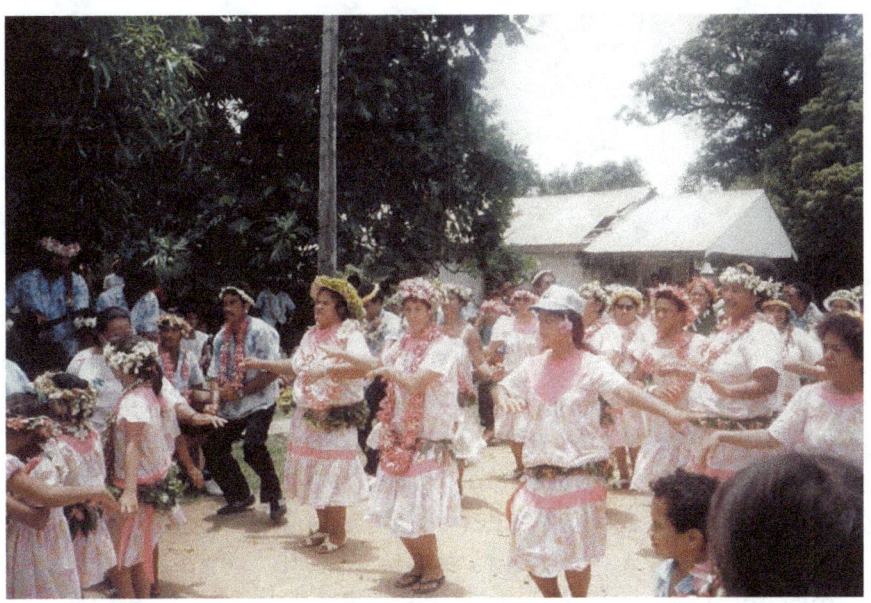

Bonita (middle of front row) dancing with local women.

24 – Ciguatera and Circumcisions

One rainy evening, an insistent knocking on our kitchen door drew us into another daunting learning curve. When I answered it, I found one of our *papa'a* friends, Ewan on the doorstep holding an islander baby boy who lay limply in his arms: his skin was pale and his head lolled unnaturally with semi-consciousness. It was a distressing sight and signalled the need for urgency.

'Mike, it's Ewan – we need your help straight away,' I called out loudly.

Mike hurried in and, taking one look at the baby, immediately grabbed the car keys and headed out through the door to drive them straight to the hospital.

In the operating theatre, Mike set-up intravenous fluids for the baby while listening to our friend's account of what had happened.

'Mana is just four months old and he's been vomiting for a few hours and pulling his legs up as if he's in bad pain.'

'Yes, he looks quite dehydrated.' Mike sped up the rate of the IV line. 'How come you're the one bringing him in? I'd have thought his family would be here.'

'Mm – well, Mana is my wife's relative, and his father's only twenty-three. He's really *akama* – you know, ashamed – because in their family, they think you must be a bad parent if your kid gets sick.' He shook his head with frustration. 'I know it doesn't make sense, but it's the way some people still think.'

'Has anyone else in the family been vomiting too?'

'Yeah, actually a few of them, I think,' Ewan replied; 'Mana's mother, Pipi's been throwing up and getting stomach pains.'

Half an hour later, when Pipi arrived at the hospital by motorbike, she was rubbing her arms and complaining of hot stinging from her ride through the rain. She also doubled over with abdominal cramps while Mike questioned her. It seemed likely that she and several other family members had developed ciguatera, a type of food poisoning, after eating a catch of mullet several hours earlier.

Ciguatera was caused by eating infected fish, and it led to vomiting, abdominal pain, diarrhoea and a strange neurological phenomenon called 'hot-cold reversal,' where cold water felt hot and vice versa.

'The rain feels hot on your skin, huh?' Mike asked and the young woman nodded miserably.

'Yeah, and I've had vomiting and belly pain for a few hours too.'

'Mm, I think it's something called ciguatera poisoning,' Mike explained and Ewan translated; 'Did you give some fish to Mana?'

The young mother shook her head in response. 'No, he's

just on breast still. I try to give him more feeds, but he just keep throwing up.'

She looked confused and guilty, but Mike assured her that she had done her best and encouraged her for trying. He was puzzled at this unusual presentation.

Ciguatera was a curious condition caused by an unusual train of events. When small marine creatures fed on damaged coral, they produced a toxin that passed into the fish that ate them. The toxin remained within affected fish even with cooking, freezing or processing; in fact, it was so stable that it became more concentrated along the food chain. From time to time, as with Pipi's family, we had seen people on the island who'd accidentally eaten toxic fish because they had looked and tasted perfectly normal, unlike other kinds of food poisoning. However, this was the first time that Mike had heard of ciguatera being transmitted through breastmilk. Given the stability of the toxin though, he reasoned that it was certainly possible.

'I think that this ciguatera poison has gone through the breastmilk to the baby, so now his guts can't work properly till it leaves his system,' Mike explained to Pipi, 'It's like there's a blockage in his bowel called an "ileus." We need to give him water into his blood like this, until he gets better.' He shook the plastic tubing as Ewan translated for the young woman.

Pipi looked nervous. 'Does Mana need operation or go to Raro?'

Mike considered her question for a few moments. Although ciguatera was the most likely culprit, it was possible that at his young age, Mana could have developed another problem called an intussusception. This occurred when the bowel wall inverted inside itself and blocked off the central passage, leading to a bowel obstruction that sometimes required a surgical repair.

'Well, it might be best if you go with him to Raro Hospital

tomorrow on the plane,' Mike said after a pause, 'He probably just needs to be looked after there, until he stops vomiting and his guts get back to normal. But there are some other serious things that could be going on with Mana, so it would be better if they check for those in Raro.'

Erring on the safe side was always a good rule of thumb, especially with such a young infant and our lack of back-up options on the island. So Pipi and Mana went on the morning flight to Raro Hospital the following day, and we waited with interest to see what eventuated.

We later heard from Ewan that Mana had slowly recovered, and after several weeks of rehydration and observation that seemed to confirm that ciguatera had caused his illness, he and Pipi were discharged back to Aitutaki.

Shortly after this, we contacted OSB by letter to see if they could pass on any other information about ciguatera being transmitted through breastmilk, and they forwarded us a study that had been conducted around that time: it indicated that there had been rare but similar episodes reported in other Pacific regions. We learned a lot about ciguatera during our posting on the island, and especially from Mana's unusual presentation of this curious and complex disease.

~

Over the summer school holidays, there was an influx of peripubescent boys to Aitutaki. Like many pregnant islanders, numerous families made the bizarre choice to leave the superior health systems of Raro and New Zealand to seek out medical treatment for their boys on their birth islands, presumably for similar cultural reasons. A large number of these parents asked Mike to circumcise their sons, much to his dismay, since it was socially unacceptable in the Cooks for lads to reach manhood without having had this procedure done. Derisive sneers followed those who had not yet been circumcised – they were called *'kiri'* by their peers, referring to their foreskins, until they had gone through this rite of passage.

During our medical training, we had been taught that elective circumcisions were unnecessary for most males and could potentially lead to serious complications. Consequently, we had always counselled against this procedure being done routinely. However, Mike didn't feel he had much choice on Aitutaki, as it seemed to be the lesser of two evils: the implication was that, either he did them with sterile instruments and local anaesthetics, or family members would lop off the offending accessory with a kitchen knife!

No'a was one of the male nurses who'd had a vast experience of assisting in circumcisions, so Mike had arranged to meet him at the operating theatre one summer's afternoon to do a surgical list together.

'I think we've got eight boys to do today,' No'a said, as he checked the waiting area then referred back to his handwritten list.

'Do we have any sutures smaller than 3/0?' Mike asked, as he shuffled through the packets in a box on the theatre shelf, 'I hate using these huge anchor-lines for such tiny repair jobs.'

His hyperbole seemed wasted on the Māori however, who simply replied: 'Maybe there are some smaller ones in the dispensary, but I don't think we got any on the last boat.'

As they continued to set up the surgical trolley, No'a's face suddenly brightened.

'Hey Dr Mike, I was talking to my friend Toto in Raro, who works as assistant for a dentist there. He told me about this new anaesthetic *they* use that's better than the old stuff *we* use. He gave me some to bring over for the *kiri* jobs.'

Mike was distracted while looking for smaller sutures and grunted in reply.

'I'll get it ready to try today, huh?' No'a added.

Mike nodded as he left the room in search of other materials, hoping that there were still some more packets in the poorly stocked dispensary. When he returned, No'a had finished setting up and had draped the first patient ready for his procedure, with an opening through the clean sheet over the boy's genitals. He had also drawn up the syringe of local anaesthetic and placed it in a kidney dish, along with an unopened scalpel blade and a packet of gauze swabs.

Mike pulled on some disposable gloves and picked up the syringe, while the young lad winced in trepidation. Just before he began, Mike paused and looked meditatively at No'a for a moment.

'It was a dental nurse that gave you this anaesthetic stuff, was it?'

No'a grinned and nodded, keen to see how well the new agent worked.

'Have you still got the ampoule handy?'

No'a shrugged impatiently and handed Mike the empty vial from the kidney dish. Mike read the components carefully, despite the minute print.

'Ah, it's got Adrenaline in it, I see.'

No'a gave him an enthusiastic nod. 'Yeah, Toto said it works really good to stop the bleeding.'

'True, but there's a big problem with using Adrenaline on parts of the body that only get their blood supply from one artery,' Mike responded.

'Why does that matter?' grumbled the islander.

'Well – it cuts off all oxygen to that part of the body, so the tissue there shrivels up and dies,' Mike said firmly.

There was an awkward pause and the young patient looked anxiously from nurse to doctor and back again.

'But it's ok for the dentist.' No'a seemed to take these concerns as a personal slight and looked annoyed. Mike realised he was on delicate territory now, in more ways than one.

'Yes, it *is* ok for dentists,' he patiently agreed, 'But that's because the mouth has lots of arteries coming in from different places. The penis only has one artery, so if we make it spasm with Adrenaline –' Mike clenched his fist to demonstrate – 'The tissue there won't survive.'

'But we always get too much bleeding with the *kiri* jobs – this could work good,' No'a muttered stubbornly, still unconvinced about any possible downsides to using his preferred agent.

'But it's dangerous,' Mike pleaded, 'Would you really want to cause irreversible damage to this lad's private parts?'

Noa looked sullenly at the far wall without replying. The boy, who was overhearing this discussion as they were poised over his genitals, began to moan and tried to sit up. He seemed to think that a quick escape was the best tactic to deal with this grim scenario.

'Look, just wait here a minute – *both* of you –' said Mike, sensing that the young lad was about to do a runner.

No'a laid an enormous hand firmly on the boy's chest and pressed him back onto the table, while Mike pulled off his gloves and placed them carefully beside the instrument tray. They were far too rare and valuable to be discarded without use. He left the theatre, thinking that a visual image may succeed where verbal explanations had failed, and went out to a pile of refuse at the side of the hospital building.

Returning a few minutes later, he called No'a into an adjacent room and held up a small limp discoloured banana with a look of triumph: 'Hey No'a, what's this, huh?'

'It's *rubbish!*' No'a looked incredulous, evidently harbouring serious misgivings about his colleague's sanity.

'Yes, *yes* – and it's *just* what this lad's penis will look like if we put Adrenaline into it!' Mike said emphatically.

'Aah.' Comprehension began to dawn and it seemed that No'a was finally convinced. He nodded slowly then left the room to search for the usual anaesthetic ampoules.

Quickly disposing of the banana, Mike returned to the theatre and found the adolescent whimpering quietly and covering his genitals with both hands.

He kindly patted the young lad's shoulder and said: 'We'll look after you, mate – you don't need to worry – everything will be ok.'

Then he scrubbed up and applied his disposable gloves once again.

When No'a returned a few minutes later, with a syringe filled with the conventional anaesthetic agent, he'd resumed his habitual equanimity. He took a deep breath and announced with a dignified calm: 'Right – it's time we got started.'

~

The boys had devised a method of expressing their gratitude to Mike for rendering them socially acceptable with their peers. Prior to their surgery, they would carve some words into the sides of young watermelons and then harvest them several weeks later, following their procedures, when the fruit had grown to maturity.

We vividly remember a ute pulling up in our driveway one afternoon, and Mike recognised the young lad whose *kiri* had been under threat during the debate with No'a a fortnight earlier. Mike reminded me of the scenario in a brief whisper, as the boy climbed cautiously down from the truck, no doubt still tender from his recent procedure.

We smiled as we received his generous gift and read the message on the large ovoid fruit that he proffered to us. The engraved words poignantly and proudly read:

'Thank u Dr Browne!'

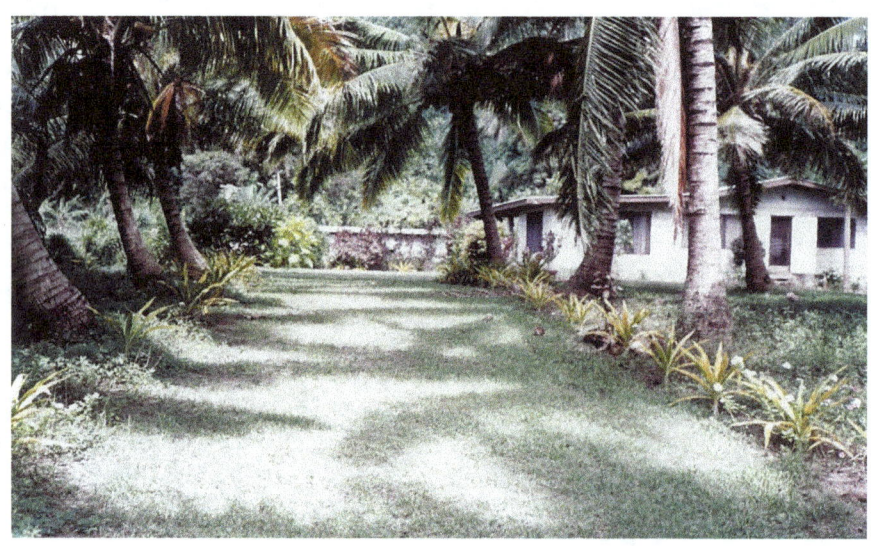

Cottage alongside Silcock's Beach.

25 – Visitors (Part II)

Aitutaki had a large lagoon that was widely considered to be one of the most beautiful in the southern hemisphere, making it a popular destination for tourists from many countries around the world. In the mid-1900s, it had been a frequent stopover point for flying-boats and, since that time, it continued to be a regular port for sea-farers on all kinds of vessels.

Many yachties visited the island to re-stock during their long sojourns across the Pacific, and we met up with some of them in the local shops as they sought out supplies and repaired their crafts. The larger boats had to anchor outside the reef, while the smaller ones sheltered in the lagoon. Occasionally, we saw medium-sized vessels tilted at steep angles by various nautical manoeuvres, so that they could traverse the shallow channel through the reef and lay anchor in the harbour.

We often invited these international visitors back to our place for a meal and to exchange tales of each other's adventures. One day, we met a pleasant Dutch couple with their six-year-old son in the general store one day and invited them home for a cuppa.

'What's your plan?' Mike asked, while their boy Erik played with our kids.

'We sold our house in Amsterdam to migrate to New Zealand,' Eduard explained, 'But instead of flying over, we decided to sail.'

Impressed by their courage and resourcefulness, I asked: 'What do you do to keep Erik entertained and educated while you travel?'

'We're home-schooling him on the boat,' replied Joanna, 'But he gets bored at times and misses the company of other children.'

She followed Erik's movements as he chased our kids around the living room. They too enjoyed having another playmate, throwing cushions across the floor at each other and laughing together. I could certainly identify with that blend of boredom, stress and loneliness that Joanna described, since it had characterised some of my own feelings during our early months on the island. In fact, I thought that having a family of three cooped up together on an eight-metre boat for six months seemed to me like a recipe for insanity.

'Come back to our place and we'll show you around,' Eduard offered at the end of their visit and we were keen to accept.

As we explored their compact vessel, we noticed that every nook was packed with the necessities of life and we praised them for their creativity. Noticing its Dutch name was PASWIND however, Mike leant over to me as we left the boat and whispered: 'I think they're really brave, but I wouldn't want to spend half a year on the open seas in a Floating Fart.'

I had to agree.

One Sunday afternoon, Mike was contacted through the hospital with a request to do a 'house call' to a ship belonging to some Italian travellers. He arrived at the wharf where they'd sent over a tender to collect him for the trip to their yacht that was anchored outside the reef. The wind was erratic and powerful, and the small motorboat tottered in the wild weather. Nausea washed over him as he pulled himself up the ladder onto the impressive thirty metre craft and a young man led him down below deck.

The ship's spectacular timber furniture, brass fittings and tasteful furnishings declared its owners to be both wealthy and keen on the comforts of life, even on the high seas. However, the fifteen passengers onboard began to outline their sufferings as soon as Mike appeared. In typical Mediterranean style, they described their symptoms with expressive charades to fill in the gaps of their English-speaking abilities. Mike diagnosed several of them as having ciguatera poisoning and discussed rehydration and anti-nauseants. They declined IV fluids but agreed to collect some medications from the hospital when they returned him to the island.

'Here, take these,' one of the women said, thrusting two silk scarves and a bundle of notes into Mike's hands as payment for his services. He tried to explain the free medical services policy of the island to them, but they waved aside his comments and ushered him back onto the tender for the squally trip back to port.

On his arrival home, Rhiannon took over the scarves to use as *pareus* (wrap-around garments) and Mike added the cash to our latest project: the 'Charge the Tourist' slush fund. We considered that since visitors to the island were usually keen to pay for any medical care we provided, the local health system should benefit in some way.

Mike counted out the notes. 'There's about one hundred New Zealand dollars here.'

Our kids wrapped up their toys in the scarves and lay them in the back of their tricycle while I looked up from folding some washing. 'Well, I noticed the last time I was in the hospital ward, the sheets looked really old and stained. We could buy about six flat sheets and some new towels for the hospital with that amount.'

Mike nodded. 'It's better than ordering them through Raro and waiting a year for them to arrive. Now that I think of it, it's been over nine months since we requested some batteries for the ambulance torches, too – we could buy some of those while we're at it.'

I nodded in agreement. 'I must say, I like avoiding these ridiculous waiting times and just buying what we need when we need it. It's much more satisfying than the usual supply – or lack of supply – system.'

We gave each other a knowing smile.

~

A steady stream of Australian friends visited us throughout our posting, mostly couples with youngsters of similar ages to our kids. We often secured furnished local houses for them to rent, although home-owners were often reluctant to commit to their properties being available until a day or two before our friends arrived – a pattern that gave rise to considerable stress for all the *papa'as* concerned. We had discovered that forward planning didn't seem to feature highly in the psyche of most locals.

We were glad to meet the Vandermoezels in person in May 1989, when they returned to Aitutaki for a fortnight's visit. They stayed with a local family that they knew well and we enjoyed sharing tales of each other's experiences of living and working on the island. Although it was the first (and only) time that we had met up, our common backgrounds and stories made us feel that we had been friends for a long time, and we've continued to stay in touch occasionally since that time.

Mike's parents, Mac and Ena returned to Aitutaki for eight weeks from March to May '89, so they were able to join in Rhiannon's fourth birthday in April and Thomas' second in May. They helped us out with minding our kids from time to time as well, including a three-day stint in which Father Luke and I did the scuba diving course with Ned – something that we both enjoyed tremendously.

On this visit, Mac and Ena spent most of their stay in the small cottage at Silcock's Beach. We loved to visit them there with its simple furnishings, overhanging pandanus palms and pawpaws loaded with fruit. We'd arrive with a picnic lunch and towels, and wander along the broad leafy path that led from their place down to the beach, as the sun sparkled through the trees and the brilliant white sand sloped into the warm blue-green water. Afternoons spent lazing in the shallows, snorkelling or paddling were all pleasurable changes from our work routine and were invariably delightful and refreshing.

On these and other outings, Thomas insisted on bringing a collection of items with him that he called his 'cow catching kit.' This included a pair of gardening gloves, a toy saw, a piece of string and a set of kitchen tongs in a small yellow plastic bucket. How he intended to use these implements to 'catch cows' was never quite clear – and what he planned to do with the beasts once he'd overpowered them was even more of a mystery. But he seemed to feel imbued with a sense of confidence, as he strode boldly along the bush tracks, with his kit always at the ready, should the contingency ever arise. Fortunately for all concerned however, it didn't.

Occasionally, Rhiannon stayed overnight with her grandparents and took on the role of tourist director with great enthusiasm. Wherever she went, she gave an all-inclusive running commentary of island life, whether anyone was listening or not.

'You must remember to have your fluoride drops each morning after breakfast,' she said, 'And when Mum and Dad give me worm tablets, I like to chew them slowly because that keeps the worms off my teeth.'

Ena smiled indulgently. 'Right, well thank you, darling – we'll try to remember that.'

When Bonita had left the island in January 1989, we had purchased her Honda 90 motorbike from her to lend to our various visitors. Mac had only ever driven a car however, so transitioning to a motorbike proved to be difficult. He also needed to get the appropriate vehicle licence, so Mike accompanied him to the police station to arrange for this several days after their arrival. As usual, it was a distinctly Polynesian affair.

'Do you have an Australian driver's licence, Mr Browne?'

'Yes.'

'Good. And do you have an Australian motorbike licence?'

'No.'

'Mm. Do you know how to ride a motorbike?'

'No.'

'Ah...'

'But I'm going to learn. My son is going to teach me.'

'Oh, well that's alright then – no problem. Here's your motorbike licence.'

'Thanks.'

'Remember: ride on the left, watch where you're going and don't fall off.'

All sorted, without the official even stepping out from behind the counter. Surprisingly, the motorbike's registration also proved to be equally informal. For a country that regularly ran aground if paperwork was not adequately completed in triplicate, the motor vehicle licensing authorities were remarkably *laissez-faire* about road safety – an issue that they appeared to consider quite trivial.

Once again, my in-laws' visit was a good excuse to indulge in various papa'a fantasies such as attending the lavish buffet brunch at the Akitua Resort. Mike happened to see three staff members for follow-up consults while we were there on one of these occasions, so our working life continued to intrude on our family time. We later introduced our relatives to Rino's for fast food, milkshakes and lemonade, that Thomas pronounced 'eleven-eight.' This outing also proved to be quite memorable, as our young son roamed from one disaster to another: losing his thongs, falling into a drain three times, finding a rotten breadfruit and smearing it all over himself, getting drenched with an outside tap, being bitten by the shop's cat, vomiting his milkshake and knocking over the 'Take Away Food' sign twice. It was an impressive effort, even by his usual standards.

Work remained the consistent backdrop of our lives, demanding our attention and energy so unerringly that it was never far from our minds. Among the many conditions that we treated, respiratory infections were common, and a surprising number of people had severe life-threatening asthma, including Rhiannon. Rather paradoxically, Mike's asthma improved while we were on the island, but recurred when we returned home, so it seemed that other factors such as local pollens and allergens must have played a part in the disparate progress of his condition.

We often saw many children between the ages of one and five years who were anaemic and malnourished. This was partly because of the islander tendency, even in their own homes, to feed small children on leftovers. Although Māori were very fond of babies, passing them from adult to adult with warm affection, once they were mobile (and possibly another sibling was on the way), toddlers were often left to their own devices. Supervision was generally quite casual and often done by older children, teens or a succession of extended family members. So, one way or another, young children were quite vulnerable to neglect.

Local kids commonly developed large painful abscesses in their necks and axillae also. To treat them, we anaesthetised the children with intramuscular Ketamine, then incised deeply into the scarlet swellings with a scalpel. The copious reeking pus sometimes burst out with such force that it slapped us in the face – a truly horrible experience. The largest abscess that Mike ever tackled was twenty-five centimetres (ten inches) across the back of an elderly Māori man, who had clearly ignored it for months. Mike took him outside the Outpatients department and doused him down with the fire-hose to remove the massive volume of stinking exudate. He suggested afterwards that we should use our 'slush fund' to invest in some hospital-supplied gumboots for wading through such extreme cases!

~

With toilet-training in progress during his grandparents' visit, Thomas insisted on trialling every lavatory available wherever we went. This infringed considerably on our attempts to relax on these outings, as we often ended up lurking around restrooms or backyards waiting for him to complete his lengthy, and usually unnecessary, ablutions. It felt rather voyeuristic, to say the least.

On the home front, Rhiannon took on her big-sisterly role by encouraging him in these endeavours as well. After he had peed into his potty, they would stand arm-in-arm, gazing in wonder and silent filial delight as the amber fluid was emptied, then shared a hug of affirmation and a round of applause together as we flushed the loo. It was a very touching scene.

On one occasion, after Thomas had fallen into a muddy puddle, Rhiannon kindly washed his clothes in a bucket and hung them on a line that she'd contrived outside the laundry. Meanwhile, I lifted him into the bath for a quick rinse, when a ten-centimetre (four inch) centipede came slithering up through the plughole towards his feet. I shrieked loudly and quickly scooped him out of the tub, then scurried off to find something heavy to dispose of this latest menace. We all viewed the bath outlet with deep suspicion after this and usually kept a brick handy and the plug *in situ*.

The island's huge centipedes wrapped themselves around unwary feet before delivering excruciating stings, so they were justifiably feared – and unlike most of the visitors that we had in our home, they were definitely of the rare but highly unwelcome variety.

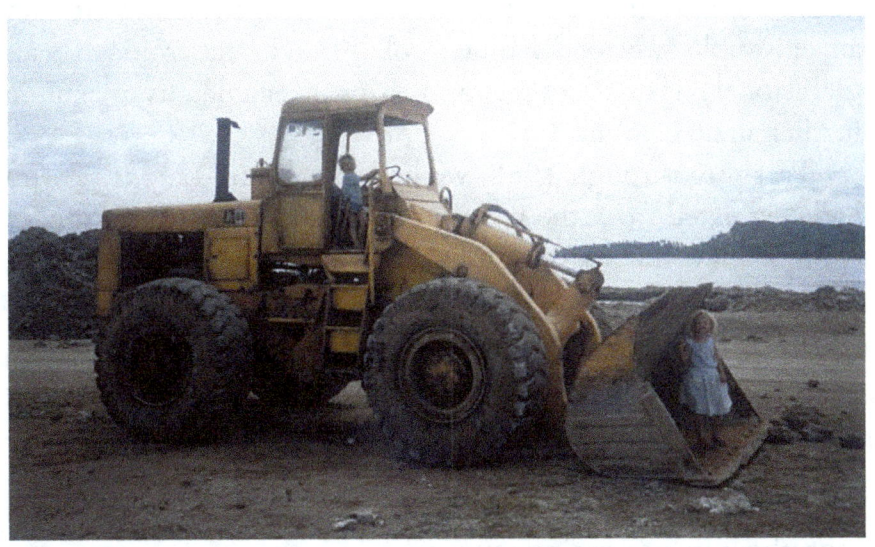

Thomas driving a 'hooge 'normous digger' with Rhiannon in the shovel.

26 – Fishing and Findings

Given our proximity to the beautiful beaches on Aitutaki, our free time was often spent around the water: swimming, snorkelling, paddling and sharing picnics with visitors, neighbours or friends. It made for easy entertainment and an enjoyable way of keeping cool through the tropical heat. Occasional trips with others in their boats enabled us to explore further afield as well.

Part-way through 1988, we had met Ewan – a *papa'a* who had originated from the UK, but had spent much of his life on Aitutaki. He was married to a local woman called Kara, and they had two daughters: seven-year-old Jane and two-year-old Tina. We all got on very well together and often helped each other out, making our friendship with them both practical and pleasant.

Ewan offered to take us on a *motu* trip one Saturday morning on one of our weekends off and we helped him to prepare his motorboat before setting out.

'Don't forget your sandals,' I called out to Rhiannon. She

ran back to rummage through our bags and we found the kids' plastic footwear. After fastening theirs on, I adjusted my own as well.

We had been warned by the Vandermoezels about the risk of serious stings and ulcers caused by standing on the back (dorsal) fins of stonefish. Our colleagues had advised us to always wear waterproof shoes on beach trips to prevent such injuries. Stonefish, as their name implied, were remarkably well camouflaged as they often had bits of seaweed attached to their surfaces and tended to burrow beneath the sandy floor of the lagoon.

'I was thankful not to get a bad injury last week,' Mike said to Ewan, as he tossed his gear into the boat.

'Yeah, what happened?'

'I was about to go out for a dive with Ned, so I didn't bother to put on my beach shoes,' he said, 'And while I stood in the water next to his boat, I felt this thing wriggle under my foot.'

'Sounds creepy,' laughed Ewan.

'Yeah, definitely,' Mike nodded, 'Fortunately it was just the side and not the dorsal fin of a stonefish, or I'd still be in agony.'

'You sure would,' Ewan agreed as he lifted his daughters into the boat; 'They're cunning little beasts that are hard to spot. I trod on one a few years ago and ended up with a horrible ulcer for weeks. It was one of the most painful things I've ever had.'

We all climbed aboard and sped through the water out to Rapota, one of the smaller *motus*, for a picnic lunch. After unpacking our gear, the kids climbed the stunted palms and Ewan showed us how to thatch a small pandanus shelter called an *are-nikau*. A cooling sea breeze ruffled the water and played across the sand as we pulled out our masks and goggles.

Snorkelling in the lagoon was splendid, as brilliant tropical fish of all sizes and colours wove in and out through the dazzling sun-sparkled waters. The lagoon floor was just as clearly visible no matter how far from shore we swam. Rhiannon and Jane were so absorbed by the scenery through their goggles that they forgot how deep the water was and kept plunging back under the surface for another enchanting view. Mike and I took turns to mind Thomas at the water's edge, or to snorkel with the others. It was hard to drag ourselves away, but we started to feel hungry and headed back to the shore around midday.

As we pulled out our sandwiches and fruit, Ewan offered to get some *nu*, and adroitly clambered up a tall palm, returning with five large green coconuts. Mike tried to imitate his technique, but like so many things, it was much harder to do than it looked. He ended up with some impressive grazes down his inner thighs and had no coconuts to show for them either. The kids giggled at his antics as they sat down under the shelter for lunch.

When we had finished eating, I suggested we see how long it took us to circumnavigate the tiny islet. We pulled on our hats and sandals and started out. Mike carried Thomas on his shoulders and he proceeded to pull hard on his father's hair.

Mike shook his head with annoyance. 'Hey, leave it off, will you?'

Thomas was in fits of wild laughter and proceeded to pull harder, so Mike put him down on the sand and he had to run to keep up with us. It took us about twenty minutes to get back to our starting point and by then the wind was becoming quite gusty.

'Time to pack up, I think,' I suggested as we gathered our gear into the beach bags and got ready to head for home.

'Let's set up some fishing lines,' Ewan said as we climbed into the boat; 'And we'll trawl on the way back. It's time to disprove the old Māori saying that *'Papa'as can't catch fish'* once and for all!'

As we travelled through the choppy waters, one of the fishing lines suddenly fell off the back of the boat. Ewan shouted in dismay and slowed the boat down to try to retrieve it, but it had disappeared into the water and we had to continue on without it. Despite this, we succeeded in catching six large silvery trevally with the other lines.

When we thanked our friend for our day-trip, we offered to buy him a replacement rod and bring over a cake during the week ahead – it was a fitting conclusion to such a fun day out on the beautiful lagoon.

One night, Ewan invited Mike to go lobstering with him on the distant reef. While they motored out, our friend took the opportunity of regaling Mike with tales of his sea-faring exploits, including the inevitable yarn of 'the one that got away.' He told how he had gone deep-sea fishing a few years earlier and had hooked an exceptionally large marlin far out to sea. It had succeeded in pulling him and his boat around for four hours before finally escaping by snapping the fifty-pound line on the motorboat's propeller: a fierce competition on both sides apparently, but it seemed the monstrous fish had won the day on that occasion.

Once they reached the reef, the two friends speared some good-sized parrotfish and found several enormous lobsters. Mike brought one home that weighed over three kilograms: I'd never seen such a huge crustacean before.

'It's too big to fit into our frypan – what'll we do with it?' I asked.

'I'll toddle up to the hospital kitchen,' Mike suggested, 'I'm sure they'll have a big pan we can borrow.'

Indeed they did, and the creature was truly delicious once cooked – we even used the remnants to make an especially gourmet soup as well. It was strange how our intake on the island varied between concoctions of tinned food or leftovers on the one hand, and rare meals fit for royalty on the other – it was simply a matter of using whatever we could lay our hands on.

The giant lobster came at some personal cost however, as Mike discovered on his return that his wedding ring had slipped off in the cool water near the reef and was gone forever. Not only that, but he sustained a deep coral cut to his foot, despite wearing his beach shoes. He required several days off work and multiple painful antibiotic injections before he fully recovered. Being the fisher, hunter and seafood gatherer for his family came with its own particular pain and loss, it seemed.

~

Once we had both learnt to scuba dive, it was a special way for Mike and me to spend our time off together, when the occasional opportunity arose and we had someone to mind our kids. Ewan took a group of us for a trip outside the reef one morning, while Rhiannon and Thomas stayed with his family for the day. It was our first dive without Ned to instruct us, so we had to pay more attention than usual to depths, times and navigation. Three men were line-fishing from the boat overhead, while a medical student called Max, Mike and I were scuba diving.

The windy wet weather made little difference to those of us below the surface; in fact, we were enjoying the thrill of hearing the distinctive calls of whales nearby. However, apart from Ewan who never got sea-sick, the squally conditions caused a good deal of vomiting for the other two above us, who produced large quantities of quality burley for the fishing!

Below the waves, the outcrops of coral started to resemble one another after a while and we became quite disorientated. When we finally re-surfaced, we found ourselves about three hundred metres from the boat and had to swim hard against the powerful currents to catch up with the others.

'Wow, that was amazing scenery,' I said when we reached the boat, 'And the whale calls were awesome.'

'It's the best live coral I've ever seen,' added Max, our diving companion, as he and I passed our tanks to Ewan and climbed back onboard.

'I think I'll snorkel here for a bit and do some spear-fishing,' Mike shouted over the noise of the wind, and he passed his tank back to us; 'There's likely to be plenty to see.'

He had succeeded in shooting three parrot-fish while snorkelling near the surface and was aiming for a fourth, when a five-foot black-tipped reef shark swam into view. Although these sharks were not generally interested in humans, they were quick to respond to a possible easy meal when they detected the 'screams' of smaller fish that were speared.

'Hey Mike,' Ewan shouted, 'Look's like you've got some company. I think I'd be getting out of there if I were you, hey?'

Mike nodded and passed up the spear-gun to Max. As he hoisted himself into the boat, the rest of us were diverted by the sight of a whale surging through the water about a hundred metres away and watched its heaving progress with great excitement. Mike stepped onto a rusty fish hook on the floor of the boat as he took off his fins and gave a sharp cry of pain; but his distress was missed by the rest of us in the general distractions caused by the whale. He bled profusely and, when I realised that the cut was quite deep, I found a rag and tied it around his foot to stem the flow.

The wind picked up further and the choppy conditions tossed us around in the motor boat. I sensed a writhing nausea within me and was keen to get started.

'Time to go, I think,' Ewan announced and pulled hard on the anchor line, but it refused to budge. He groaned with dismay. 'Oh boy, this isn't good. We need a volunteer to go back down and untangle the anchor-line if we've got any hope of getting home. I only bought that rope a month ago and I don't want to cut it off and lose it.'

He stared pointedly at the three of us who were already wet from our dive: it was clear he had no intention of jumping in himself. We all peered into the water where there were now five reef sharks encircling the boat – not an appealing sight. I stared at Mike and he stared at Max, but no one was immediately forthcoming – a stalemate in the rollicking vessel.

'Oh alright, I'll go,' Mike conceded. The rest of us gave a small cheer of relief. Pulling on his mask, fins and tank, he rolled backwards off the boat and descended down the anchor-line while the sharks disappeared from view. I found the wait a long and anxious one, as I watched to see if there was any evidence of blood or body parts floating to the surface.

Thankfully Mike was still intact when he reappeared after disentangling the reluctant anchor, and he clambered back into the boat. We were all grateful to have him safely onboard and the boat released for the homeward trip.

Unfortunately, soon after we arrived on shore, Mike's foot became severely infected from the fishhook injury and he developed lymphangitis and a tender swollen groin. The infection was too widespread for oral antibiotics to work, and it was only following three days of deep intramuscular Penicillin that his symptoms finally settled. Once his butt hurt more than his foot, he decided the infection had rounded the corner enough to ease off with the painful daily jabs!

I've always been very thankful that both Mike and I had learned to scuba dive during our time on Aitutaki: it was an intriguing interface between the daily challenges of our life and work on the island, and the idyllic natural world beyond it. Our instructor Ned was a great teacher and generous with his invitations for us to go with him, if he had spare seats on his boat, when one or occasionally both of us were able to join in.

'I don't like all the drivel the tourists go in for,' Ned moaned to Mike one day; 'I just want to take them out, bring them back and pocket the cash without the "Oh, what fish is that – it's all so amazing" crap day after day.'

Mike sympathised: 'Yes, I can imagine it gets pretty monotonous.'

Ned suddenly brightened up. 'Actually, if you'd be prepared to do the talking on the boat and wash off the gear when we get back, I'd be happy to give you and Michele cheap dives whenever I've got spare seats.'

'Definitely!'

Mike was able to do enough of these dives to qualify for his advanced NAUI certificate by the time we left the island, and we both appreciated the opportunities to escape from our constant and unpredictable work demands into such spectacular scenery so close at hand.

Aitutaki is still rated among the top five dive sites in the world due to its 95% live coral, abundant tropical fish, year-round water temperature of 26 degrees Celsius and 100+ foot visibility. Like all coral atolls, the mainland of Aitutaki was simply the tip of a prehistoric volcano and the *motus* were adjacent smaller peaks. The outer reef was absolutely stunning and beyond the coral, the 'drop-off' appeared, as the sides of the volcanic mountain plunged steeply downwards into the inky darkness of the sea.

When diving near the drop-off, I found it disconcerting to consider that, since the ocean was over four kilometres (2.5 miles) deep at this point, it could have contained any number of ancient and gigantic creatures. After all, these seas were beyond the reach of scientists then, and even now hold many mysteries, due to the challenges of probing such incalculable depths.

On one occasion, Mike and I were diving together where the slanting light began to dissipate into the vast ocean. At around seventy feet, I suddenly nudged Mike as I saw an enormous sting-ray circling up from the drop-off towards us. Its wingspan was at least four metres – a terrifying sight as it moved closer to us with every steady beat. It seemed to look towards me with a curious kind of detachment and I stopped kicking and tried to keep as still as possible. I figured that if I could try to imitate a rock-form rather than a human, it may lose interest and go away. Whatever the reason, I was greatly relieved when it resumed the rhythmic movement of its massive wings, then slowly and silently disappeared from view.

Nothing can really describe the sublime exploration of this eerie exotic place around the reef: the immense and vivid underwater garden. Rolling and writhing in the dappled sun-split liquor of this primeval womb, we were suspended above vast platters of coral that seethed with countless brilliant whorls of fish, pulsating with life-forms, the intricate kaleidoscope of colours and shapes ceaselessly weaving down and up, out and in, light and shadow, immersed in such warm and weightless watery depths of exuberant fecundity.

Truly – it was bliss.

In mid-August, the winds tended to come from a more westerly direction onto the island, creating the rare opportunity of snorkelling or diving outside the eastern side of the reef. Even Ned, who'd explored numerous areas around Aitutaki for decades, had only been able to dive in this region on several occasions, making it a truly unique part of the reef and indeed, the planet.

In August 1989, Ned invited Mike to go diving with him in this region. Although the ocean looked relatively calm on this particular day, the swells were thirty feet high making it potentially quite perilous. Even at a depth of seventy feet, the surging currents were powerful and irresistible.

Exploring this part of the reef was exhilarating, with superb corals and a super-abundance of fish and sea-life. While at a depth of sixty feet, Mike came across an enormous conch shell in perfect condition – it was about the same size as a soccer ball and would have made a great souvenir or sold for quite a price. But when Mike saw the creature's head slowly emerge from the trumpet-shaped opening, with its two yellow, snail-like eyes looking into his own, he felt deeply chastened. It would have been sheer treachery to take this magnificent creature from its home for the sake of having a trophy he reasoned, and he reverently replaced it onto the nearby rocky platform.

In a final salute, the two exchanged a long look of enquiry and acknowledgement, before Mike grasped the anchor line and, admiring a myriad of other untouched delights, he slowly ascended from this vast and silent swaying secret garden.

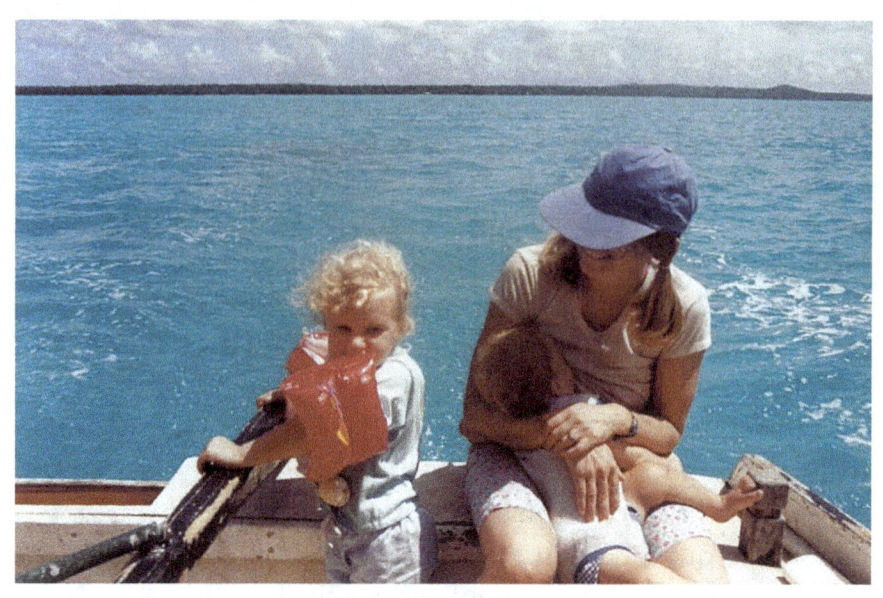

Michele & kids on *motu* trip. Thomas breastfeeding *again!*

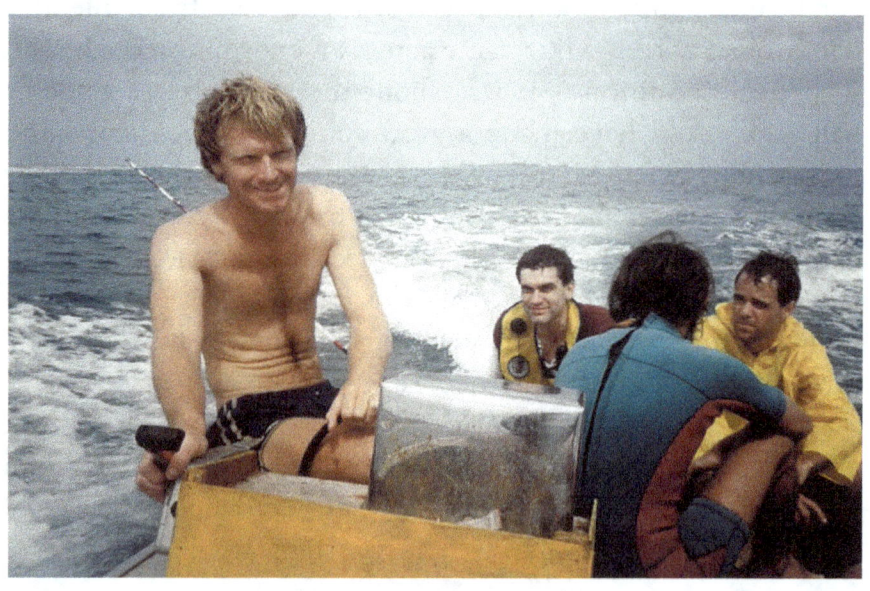

Ewan (far left) with Mike & volunteer friends going on a fishing trip.

27 – Repairs and Relief

In July 1989, Dr Rua went to Rarotonga for a fortnight to attend the 24th Anniversary commemorations of Constitution Week. His absence meant that we assumed the management of all medical services on the island once again.

At the same time, we received a telegram from Raro Hospital announcing that the following afternoon, the New Zealand ophthalmology team whom we had met previously, were returning to the island for several days. This included the surgeon Dr Jeffrey, his wife Moira and the optometrist, Hamish. We had to find accommodation for them and round up any relevant patients, as no eye services had been available since their previous visit eighteen months earlier. Getting all this sorted with less than 24 hours' notice created considerable stress, on top of the 24/7 medical cover that we were already providing.

The Kiwis arrived on a Friday afternoon and we met them at the airport with a box of *eis* rapidly constructed by the hospital staff. We decided to take them to the Rapae for Island Night, as this was the easiest way to feed them on their arrival, and after dinner, Mike drove them to the hospital for an evening of consulting.

Saturday morning began with four cases requiring cataract surgery, and once again, Mike gave the anaesthetics while Moira assisted her husband. Hamish did eye assessments on the school kids who had missed out on their checks when the team had visited previously. Over the remainder of their stay, we hosted them for various meals and arranged a lagoon trip on Saturday afternoon. Rhiannon kept Moira amused by teaching her Preschool medleys and Māori dance routines.

When we took the team to the airport on Monday afternoon, Thomas pulled off his shorts and mounted the flagpole podium, where he provided some spontaneous entertainment by peeing into a crowd of tourists. During this display, his tiny underpants blew over the fence onto the end of the runway and he ran around the barricade to retrieve them – thankfully without endangering life or limb. After our intense weekend of multi-tasking, we were glad that it had all ended with a moment of comic relief and not in tears!

~

In the second half of 1989, petrol supplies to the island ran out for many weeks, resulting in major problems for everyone. The inter-island transport ship, the MV Manuvai, had run aground in late 1988 and, since it had been the only vessel that had ferried the 200-litre (forty four gallon) drums of petrol to Aitutaki and returned the empty ones to Raro for refilling, there were no longer consistent fuel supplies on the island.

As a result, all was strangely quiet: mowers, vehicles and motor boats had mostly ground to a halt, rendering many common pursuits such as mowing and fishing difficult for everyone. Fortunately, we had a spare thirty litre container of petrol for our own car, so we were still mobile, but we had to be as frugal as possible with our trips, since we didn't know how long the fuel-drought would continue.

Meanwhile, both hospital ambulances were dying by degrees and there was no likelihood of the Department of Health replacing them until they'd completely expired. Consequently, maintaining the function of the ambulances became almost as much of a hospital priority as keeping the patients alive.

Our own vehicle, Hilda, required a certain amount of attention too, with points and plugs, shock absorbers and other car parts brought over by various Aussie visitors. Ned taught Mike how to paint the wheel bays, boot, vehicle under-sides and inside of the doors with diesel oil to slow down the inexorable rusting process. We also touched up spots of damaged duco with nail polish, as this virulent process began within hours of exposure to the salty elements on the island.

~

During our posting, we had had some tortuous encounters with the Public Works Department, so we had learnt to send in requests for repairs with very low expectations of either timely or quality workmanship.

Our bathroom had had no basin when we arrived and several months after our request for one, the department had sent over a few plumbers in their trade-mark blue overalls, who soon had a stained recycled bowl attached to the bathroom wall. We were just getting used to cleaning our teeth over this receptacle, instead of spitting into the bath, when it crashed into pieces on the floor, narrowly missing the kids' toes.

Second time around, our request for repairs resulted in an

even longer wait, until eventually a few more workers appeared with another stained recycled bowl. Presumably they had used dyna-bolts as well as concrete this time, as the basin remained attached to the bathroom wall for the remainder of our stay – it was a gratifying outcome by usual Public Works standards.

However, I was quite distressed when our ancient wringer washing machine ground to an ear-piercing stop one day and I had to call the Public Works Department yet again to get this appliance repaired. It took two months for any action and this prolonged period of hand-washing did little to improve our work-life balance in the interim.

Eventually however, a team of eight workmen arrived one afternoon – a large number of technicians to attend to a single piece of machinery, I thought. But I wasn't going to ask awkward questions, since I was desperate to have this essential service restored as soon as possible.

I knew well enough by then that supplying food to tradesmen in any and every culture was always advantageous, so I had brought in platters of watermelon to spur them on in their endeavours. It was rather disheartening therefore, to return a few hours later, only to find them all sitting on the laundry floor alongside the untouched machine, with a desultory Māori conversation being the sole activity in evidence.

'Is there a problem?' I enquired politely, not wishing to get them off-side.

They had obviously decided the best approach was to bamboozle me with technical jargon.

'Mm, well we need a Phillip's head screwdriver, Mrs Dr Browne,' the self-appointed spokesman explained.

'Well, actually we've got one of those.' I brightened up and went to find the necessary item in our toolbox. Their faces fell when I presented it to them with an enthusiastic flourish.

Grumbling in disconsolate tones, they struggled to their feet.

'Ah, well we need some ... other things too,' the tradesman added, as they all ambled out through the doorway.

'When will you be back?' I pleaded, but their retort was an unintelligible mumble. I had interrupted their downtime and they were tetchy, to say the least.

As the delay in repairs continued with no end in sight, Mike decided to tackle the problem himself with the assistance of one of our *papa'a* friends. Since Steve had spent much of his working life repairing plane engines and propellers, a washing machine was relatively small fry for him. *(Why didn't we think to ask him sooner?)*

The two men sawed up some bits of old steel pipe, welded them to the original drive shaft and had the machine working again within a few hours. Oh, such joy!

~

Bonita's departure from Aitutaki in January '89 had left a huge hole in our lives, and we missed our regular sharing of day-to-day life with her over countless comforting cups of tea.

So we were delighted to make some new friends in April '89, especially when we learned that they planned to stay on the island for four months. Sam and Rachel Stephens were Kiwis in their mid-fifties and their adult kids and assorted grandchildren lived back in New Zealand. They moved into the small unit block that Bonita had previously occupied. Stan was a retired headmaster and he had taken up a part-time position doing relief teaching at the local high school. We also welcomed them to our regular Tuesday night group along with Father Luke.

As we chatted over supper one evening, Sam asked: 'What's been one of the most difficult aspects of your time on Aitutaki?'

Mike munched on a biscuit as he considered his answer. 'Well, for me it would have to be the sense of social disconnection from others, I think. You see, there are only about twenty *papa'as* on the island, and they're a very odd lot, you know – including us!'

Luke chuckled – we always found his gentle and thoughtful disposition so endearing. Continuing the conversation, he added. 'Yeah, I don't think most normal people would even consider coming here for an extended period, so I guess that means we're all rather "different" by definition.'

'Yep,' Mike said with a smile, 'So there are very few *papa'as* that we can be really honest with about what we're going through – especially the work difficulties, but also things like when our kids get sick.'

'I agree,' I nodded, 'And because we're the only *papa'a* health workers here, there aren't any other people who feel the same high highs when patients recover, or low lows when they don't, or our frustrations when the supplies don't arrive – things like that. The hospital staff have very different attitudes from us, so we don't feel like we can debrief with them in the same way that we could with colleagues back home, for instance.'

'And anyway, you have to be careful if you moan to the locals here,' Luke added, 'Because they're all related to each other. You might end up saying the wrong thing to the wrong person if you don't watch out!'

'Mm, dangerous,' said Rachel, pursing her lips.

I sipped my tea and rejoined: 'I also remember our predecessors, the Vandermoezels, saying to us in a letter: "You're not islanders and you never will be – so there's no point in acting like you are." At first, that seemed a rather strange and obvious thing to say, but now I think I know what they meant. Although we try to understand the Māori priorities and customs, we'll never think about life as they do, and we'll never relate to them in exactly the same way that they relate to each other.'

'Ah, so it's a different kind of isolation from just the physical distance from home?' Sam confirmed.

'Yes, absolutely,' Mike replied, 'So we can end up feeling quite lonely at times. I think we would've gone "reef-crazy," as Bonita would say, without at least a *few* people who we could really be ourselves with. So I hope you can put up with plenty of whinges or belly laughs when we get together – just remember that you're helping to save our sanity!'

Our friends laughed as they passed around the biscuits that they'd brought, and we topped up everyone's tea for the third time.

~

The Stephens were like surrogate grandparents to our kids and occasionally minded them, so that Mike and I could have rare but treasured opportunities to scuba dive together or share a meal out by ourselves. Their involvement in our lives proved to be especially valuable at times when we would otherwise have felt completely overwhelmed.

On one of these occasions, I had been busy at Outpatients all morning and then checked over some of the in-patients during the long, wet afternoon. In the middle of 1989, Mike and I had adjusted our job-sharing arrangement, as I had wanted to do more medical work than previously, and he preferred to spend more time at home with the kids. So we had alternated roles week by week: one of us did Monday to Friday at the hospital while the other was at home, and the following week we swapped. I continued with my Women's Health Clinic, and Mike still did all the obstetrics and his usual share of the afterhours load with

Dr Rua as well.

One of the midwives, Tua, called to me through the doorway of the Outpatient clinic as I was finishing for the day, 'Hey, Dr Michele, we got a mama just come to labour ward.'

'Sure,' I said, 'I'm going home now, so I'll let Dr Mike know when I get there.'

'Yeah, she's one of the mamas that he delivered last year and now she come back again with another *pepe*, huh?' She giggled with amusement.

'Ok, I'll tell him. Maybe you can send the ambulance down in about ten minutes,' I added as I headed out the door.

The torrential rain that we had been experiencing for days had turned the hospital road into a quagmire of mud and gravel, and our car slithered crazily as I drove home, bone-weary and longing for a quiet cuppa on my arrival. As I walked through the kitchen door however, I was assailed by the putrid stench of raw sewerage.

Apparently, our septic system that was erratic at the best of times, had reached a point of complete overload after three days of heavy rain, and copious effluent had poured up through our shower outlet into the bathroom and living areas.

I groaned as I took in the chaotic scene. Mike was wearing gumboots and he waved a wet broom at the stinking mess.

'It's been horrendous as you can see. The septic's overflowed and I've been trying to get it cleared up before you got home.'

'No such luck, huh?'

I heard the kids squabbling over some books as they perched on our bed. At least they were out of reach of the mess, I registered briefly.

'Sadly, no,' he replied, running a hand through his unruly hair, 'I went outside to dig around the old earthenware drains for a while. They're really choked up with weeds and roots, but

I think I've managed to clear some of the muck and they're starting to drain a bit better now. But unfortunately, the crap had already gone all over the lino by then.'

He waved his broom at the large sheets of linoleum that leant against the dining room wall, and buckets of water nearby that he'd started to use on the clumps of sewerage that stuck to the garish surfaces.

'I don't suppose you could give me a hand?' he added.

Just then, the familiar but unwelcome sound of revving came through the windows as the ambulance arrived in our driveway. I suddenly recalled the midwife's message.

'Gosh, that's right, I've just remembered – Tua told me that there's a new admission in labour ward for you. Apparently, it's one of the mamas you delivered last year, and she's come back with her second one now.'

'Oh no,' Mike groaned, 'Great timing.' He walked out to the kitchen doorstep where he swapped his stinking gumboots for his joggers. With a brief wave, he disappeared into the ute that immediately backed out of our yard.

As the kids' yells grew in volume, I crumpled onto a nearby chair, weighed down by an oppressive sense of loneliness and exhaustion. I silently prayed for aid in the grey light of the clammy afternoon.

A few moments later, there was a knock at the kitchen door and our Kiwi friends stood on the doorstep. Although I could see no evidence of 'wings,' the words 'angelic visitation' immediately sprang to mind at this remarkably timely response to my supplications.

'Oh dear – what can we do to help?' Rachel said, looking at the chaotic scene and the tears trickling down my face.

I was overwhelmed with gratitude. 'Gosh, would you really want to? It's *so* disgusting.' The foul smell was quite overwhelming. 'If you could take the kids back to your place for a while, that would be brilliant.'

She tiptoed through the puddles to the bedroom. We carried one child each out to our car and I passed over the keys for her to drive them home to their unit. By the time I turned back to the disaster that was our living room, Sam had already set to work with buckets, hose, brooms and mop, and we worked steadily together for the next few hours.

At last, we gave a small cheer – order had finally been restored and the malodorous muck was gone. I washed my hands and put on the kettle for a much-needed pot of strong tea and sweet biscuits, as we sank gratefully onto the cane lounge-chairs. Rachel returned with the kids a short time later – they were all in good spirits, having enjoyed some snacks and games together.

I made them an offer that I hoped they'd both accept: 'Would you like to stay for dinner? Someone dropped in a big trevally last night, so there's plenty to share. And anyway, it's the least I can do after all your help today. I don't know how I would've survived without you both…'

I wiped some tears from my cheeks as the kids hugged my legs.

'Well, only if you're sure.' Sam looked to Rachel for confirmation.

'Yes, yes, stay with us, stay with us,' the kids chanted and Rachel smiled back and nodded.

Sam helped to peel some veggies as I cooked the fish in a buttery frypan, and Rachel bathed the kids. Although it was much later than usual, the meal felt like a celebration of survival. Mike joined us towards the end of dinner, following his slow but successful delivery. We even had a small serve of festive ice-cream to mark our shared sense of achievement – it lifted our spirits considerably.

We farewelled our friends with much affection after our meal that night, so grateful for their timely and good-hearted assistance.

There was a further sewerage leak with heavy rain later that night after the kids had gone to bed, but we managed to contain it by ourselves. This had been one of those horrible protracted days, when we'd both felt pushed to the limits of endurance in every possible way. Climbing back from this particular low point over the following weeks felt much longer and harder than usual.

On the phone the next morning, Mike had strong words with the Public Works Department, insisting that serious plumbing repairs needed to be done as soon as possible.

'Apparently these drains were supposed to be swapped for PVC pipes over a year ago because they're so blocked up, but it still hasn't happened,' he said; 'We're paying 15% of our income to rent this place, and we don't intend to continue our medical work here with soiled toilet paper stuck to our shoes, ok?'

'Yeah, yeah, we'll get to it.' The reply was terse and non-specific.

Unfortunately, they didn't 'get to it' – well, not before we left the island, anyway. However, although we couldn't commend the Public Works Department for their response, at least the stinking overflow was not repeated either. Along with our life-saving friends and their remarkable assistance, we continued to be thankful for this and many other small domestic mercies.

28 – Veterinary Variety

Since there was no vet on Aitutaki, Mike was sometimes co-opted into doing procedures on animals by various *papa'as*. These ventures required a high level of ingenuity and experimentation with both anaesthetics and surgery, since he'd had no prior experience with veterinary techniques. They also resulted in a further expansion of his holistic clinical skills.

Phil was a *papa'a* who sometimes helped us out with electrical and handyman repairs. One day, he called about his elderly but dearly loved cat, and asked Mike to check him over. The animal was a remarkable 14kg and was quite appropriately called Ugly. Apparently, he'd developed a strange yowling cry several days earlier after eating some *mito*, a surgeonfish with a scalpel-like ridge on its back. Phil was concerned that his pet may have damaged his throat or swallowed some bones in the process.

To investigate further, Mike thought that the best approach would be to insert the smallest of his three paediatric laryngoscopes that he had brought over from Australia. Faced with the cat's hostile glares and formidable incisors however, he decided that Ugly needed to be anaesthetised first. He elected to use a bottle of ether (circa 1950) that he'd found in a neglected cupboard in the hospital's operating theatre when cleaning it out one day.

Using this anaesthetic agent required a delicate balance of ether vapour and room air for which no precise dispensing apparatus was available, especially for an animal. So Mike experimented with pouring the ether into an ashtray that was placed next to the cat's nose, while Phil gently but firmly restrained his beloved Ugly. The creative device used to regulate the intake of ether and air was provided by placing a golf cap over the cat's head and partially over the ashtray. Judicious adjustments of the cap's peak allowed an effective titration of the gases and Ugly soon fell into a deep sleep.

Mike then inserted his laryngoscope into the feline oropharynx: it provided excellent visualisation of the animal's laryngeal region and vocal cords. No foreign body or laceration was found, so he took the opportunity of injecting a generous dose of out-of-date Penicillin into the cat's shoulder muscles. He removed the golf cap, and over time, Ugly resumed a dribbly semi-consciousness. His symptoms resolved and he was soon back to his fat happy self.

Phil was so overjoyed with this outcome that he came over to our place a fortnight later with a large slab of freshly caught tuna, about 3kgs in total. It was a win-win situation, as Ugly continued to do well and this gift of pure protein provided us with many delicious meals over the next few weeks.

~

From time to time, various *papa'as* like Ewan asked Mike to castrate their young male pigs. The reason for this was that, as they reached puberty and began to produce high levels of testosterone, boars became very lean, mean creatures indeed. Removing their testicles early in life reduced them to chubby contented beasts, and that suited their owners very well.

Since the hospital often had out-of-date drugs and suture materials, Mike found the most expired items to use for this veterinary work. While he tried to do these procedures in a clean setting, there was no possibility of sterile conditions, as they were generally done in sheds or out of doors.

Mike's technique was to anaesthetise the pig by injecting the nape of its thick neck with intramuscular Ketamine, having discovered that the porcine dose was about three times that used for humans. Once the animal was asleep, he used a scalpel to open the scrotal sac, tie off the blood vessels with catgut ligatures and remove the testicles. He then sutured the wound and allowed the animal to gradually wake up to its new and docile existence. At that time, the going 'rate for payment' was a hind quarter of pork for several castrations. This suited us very well – especially when we had forth-coming visitors or special occasions.

Another time, Mike was asked to repair a large gash down the side of a sow that had been gored by an especially violent boar. Ketamine and suturing did the job again, with a further successful (if not especially artistic) outcome.

~

One day, Mike had taken Rhiannon with him to do a home visit. Following the consultation, they heard that the family's pig was in the process of delivering a litter, so they headed out to the yard to watch the proceedings. Rhiannon was fascinated to see the squirming slippery piglets emerge one after another until there were ten in all.

Thankfully, the sow was distracted by the birthing process and consequently not troubled by our daughter's attentions as she took great delight in lining up each piglet next to its respective teat and pushing their groping mouths in the right direction. Chattering incessantly to the small creatures, she firmly restored their positions if they moved out of line and took on a role that was somewhere between a midwife and a parking attendant. Mike and the local family were amused to watch her fulfilling her new chore so diligently.

~

Since dogs were not allowed on Aitutaki, Thomas was totally oblivious of their existence in his early life. When he saw them during our brief trip to Raro in mid-1988, he thought they were pigs and snorted vigorously whenever he saw them. After our return to Australia, he discovered dogs everywhere and was terrified of them – even those that were very distant and ignoring him completely.

In contrast, plenty of stray cats roamed the island. Their lives were often far from easy however, due to the unwanted attentions of some of the less compassionate kids. A particular mama cat hung around the hospital and was well fed by us or the other staff whenever she looked hungry. One day, Mike came into our office at work to find that she'd given birth to a litter of kittens in the desk drawer. It required a bit of cleaning up, but no one seemed too fazed about the hygiene implications of the feline delivery in a consulting room.

Late in our first year, our friend Bonita had salvaged a young kitten from some unruly school students and brought her over to our house. She was a cute little tabby, probably about four weeks of age. Because of the imminent festive season, Rhiannon decided she should be called 'Christmas' or 'Smas' for short. She was so small that she couldn't lap up milk by herself, so we had to feed her with an eyedropper. Rhiannon gently wrapped her in dolls' blankets and lined her box with leaves. Thomas mewed non-stop at her, but his attempts to feed her resulted in well-intentioned but vigorous jabs with the eye-dropper to any part of her tiny torso. However, his cat imitations quickly turned to screams of terror if she started to crawl towards him: rather ironic for such a tough young guy!

Smas grew rapidly and was much enjoyed by our whole family, but she developed a dangerous habit of sleeping next to the back wheels of our car. Unfortunately, I failed to notice her there one day and ran over her. It was a traumatic situation for everyone and we had to have a burial ceremony to mark her passing. We all really missed her.

Some months later, we were donated another kitten that four-year-old Rhiannon decided to call 'Jemima Anne'.

'So, what made you think of calling her "Jemima Anne," sweetheart?' I asked.

'Well we don't *already* have a cat called "Jemima Anne," do we?' she retorted brusquely.

It wasn't quite what I'd meant – after all, we didn't already have a cat of *any* name – even *I* couldn't have missed something that was *that* entirely self-evident. But I shook my head in humble concurrence, nevertheless, and moved on to other salient aspects of pet ownership.

Jemima Anne proved to be a hardy and good-natured cat. She accepted being carried under one arm or wheeled around as the 'baby' in various games. She wasn't especially keen on Thomas's attempts to put her in our saucepans though, and quickly escaped before he could put the lids on top and trap her inside.

She had a voracious appetite too and grew remarkably quickly, until one day Rhiannon pointed at her and said: 'Will you look at the size of that scrotum?'

Yet again, she was right. We had completely misjudged the gender of our pet, and had to promptly re-name him as 'Jimmy Andy' after that.

When we were leaving the island, we were concerned about who would take on JA's care. Strays were often mistreated and we wanted him to go to a good home. Thankfully, a *papa'a* couple who had recently moved to Aitutaki to set up a business, were keen cat-lovers and happy to take him on. We dropped him off to his new owners' place during the final weeks of our posting.

When we saw him some days later, we were relieved to see that we had made the right decision. JA had wasted no time in settling into the child-free household, where his food and water bowls were always promptly replenished. We found him luxuriating on mounds of cushions and looking thoroughly content with his new life of unencumbered feline extravagance.

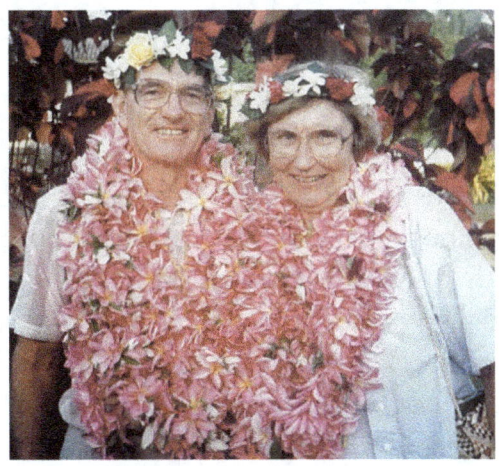

Farewell to the Stephens.

29 – Incidents and Illnesses

A large number of complex medical cases occurred in concentrated bouts from time to time during our posting, and one of these spells began with a fatal road crash in the latter half of 1989. On this occasion, a motorbike rider and his pillion passenger collided head-on at high speed with another motorcyclist on a narrow, unsealed track. High alcohol levels and the absence of helmets, that were not required by Cook Island law, probably contributed to the severity of the accident as well.

The rider of one motorbike had a massive head injury and, despite Mike's most valiant efforts, died overnight. His pillion passenger remained unconscious for twelve hours, but slowly recovered from his severe concussion and soft tissue wounds over the next few weeks. The other rider had several broken limbs and large lacerations that required painstaking suturing with our usual suboptimal materials.

The nurses were not familiar with the recommended observations for head traumas, so I wrote up a list for them of the hourly checks that they should follow over the next few days. It was another opportunity for us to upskill them with a protocol that they could, and hopefully would, use again in future head injury cases.

The responsibility of treating these seriously ill patients concurrently weighed heavily on Mike and sapped his dwindling reserves of energy. He staggered home to eat or shower every twelve hours or so, shattered and anxious, until those who survived were past the most perilous stages of their injuries. I tried to support him with long debriefs and some of his favourite meals, or swapped work shifts with him, to share the load whenever possible.

Shortly after this event, Mike responded to a phone request for a home-visit one afternoon and, for various reasons, he had two-year-old Thomas with him. He drove our car to the outskirts of Vaipeka village to attend to the injured man, as the ambulance was needed elsewhere at the time.

Twenty-year-old Ivi had fallen from a coconut tree an hour earlier and now lay on the sandy floor of the small hut where he lived with his extended family. Mike examined him in the dim light where the young man was groaning in distress. The long gash down the side of Ivi's face and his muddled speech indicated a head injury, but fortunately his trunk seemed to be reasonably intact. Mike also discovered the agonising deformities of his two badly broken wrists: he immobilised them with makeshift splints composed of sticks from the backyard and bandages from his work bag. An injection of morphine also helped to allay the worst of Ivi's sufferings.

While Mike was treating the young man, Thomas crouched on his haunches and watched the process with interest. He then noticed a baby girl on the far side of the hut, straightened up and proceeded to walk directly over Ivi's belly to investigate the infant further. As she lay on a mattress on the floor and gazed around at those in the room, she suddenly trembled with alarm as she saw Thomas towering over her.

He sat down on the mattress beside her and proceeded to pat her small belly and hum some of his favourite songs. However, he stopped suddenly when he discovered her nappy was drenched and cried out with considerable agitation: 'Wet nappy – baby's Mummy – change it!'

In his young mind, this crisis was far more compelling than that of the man he had just clambered over, and his angst continued unabated until the infant's mother responded to his demands.

Once the ambulance arrived, Mike helped to transfer Ivi onto a stretcher with the assistance of his father and the driver, and together they hauled the stretcher onto the back of the ute. Mike buckled Thomas into his car-seat, drove our car along the rough unsealed track behind the ambulance and collected me on the way past our place, while Rhiannon was playing with her friends across the road. We both plastered Ivi's fractures when we got him to the operating theatre, and shared the task of suturing and cleaning up his ragged gravelly skin-tears.

After a frustrating delay with the phone system, Mike arranged for the young man's semi-urgent transfer to Raro on a domestic flight the following day, for further investigations and treatment. Once all this was accomplished, we gathered up our roaming toddler and wearily headed for home.

~

Four-year-old Rhiannon had picked up various medical words through accompanying us on ward rounds or listening in to our conversations, and she incorporated these terms into her games:

'You'll have to have Paracetamol for that terrible cough.'

'Let's look at these eyes – mm, not too good – take these drops four times a day. Now your stomach: make sure you eat good food. Oh, that leg looks a bit broken – I'd better bandage it up.'

'This baby's been sick for two minutes – I think she needs a drip.'

While her comments were quite insightful, we were a little concerned about her tendency towards over-servicing!

One day she asked us for a more detailed description of 'how babies come out' so that she could 'play it better' with her toys. We explained things as well as we could, although our explanations had to be somewhat abridged for someone of her tender years.

As it happened, some weeks later a midwife rang up to inform Mike of an impending delivery when we were about to leave home for an evening trip out for fish and chips.

'How about we all go to the hospital this time instead of waiting for you here,' I suggested; 'Hopefully this mama will give birth quickly and we can go straight to Rino's afterwards.'

'Good plan,' Mike nodded and we all piled into the car and drove up to the hospital.

While he disappeared inside, I sat in the shady garden and chatted to Thomas as he climbed some wiry *tipani* trees, and Rhiannon wandered around collecting flowers and leaves. Half an hour soon passed and I suddenly realised that our daughter had disappeared.

'Do you know where Rhiannon is?' I asked Thomas, but he was distracted with his climbing and shrugged carelessly. A fretful anxiety gnawed inside me as I started to search the grounds, when Mike emerged from the building.

'Have you seen Rhiannon?' I asked.

Mike seemed a bit disconcerted. 'Well actually I have, though not in the way you'd think. I was just finishing the delivery when I turned around and saw her standing right behind me. She was just starting to wander out of labour ward.'

'Ah, I see.' The source of his discomfort began to dawn on me. 'Do you think she saw the delivery?'

Just at that moment, we looked up and saw her coming towards us with her hands clasped around her neck and a strangled grimace on her face.

'Mm – well, if that expression means what I think it does, then yes, she probably did,' Mike said with a grin.

I nodded in agreement and we both watched to see how affected she was by her unusual experience. Her hands dropped from her neck and she quietly resumed collecting flora.

'Ok, well it's time to go,' Mike announced and lifted Thomas off a nearby branch.

'Did you see anything interesting when you went around the hospital?' I asked our daughter as we climbed back into the car.

'Mm, yes,' she reflected; 'And I think I know how babies come out now. It's a bit yuk, though – they come out of the Mummy's *bottom*.' She shuddered with distaste.

'Uh-huh,' I replied; 'Well I guess at least you'll be able to play it properly with your toys now, hey?'

She nodded silently in response, apparently deep in thought.

Mike and I smiled at each other and resumed our evening quest for fast food by driving on to Rino's. The fish and chips were excellent with real potatoes this time, too – a rare but thoroughly enjoyable treat – and we relished every mouthful.

All things considered, the evening had proved to be quite an unconventional but memorable family night out.

The Boy Scout movement was well supported on Aitutaki with enthusiastic participants keen to learn new skills. One of the leaders approached Mike at Outpatients one day and asked: 'Mr Dr Browne, would you be able to run an exam for our scouts for their First Aid Certificates?'

'What have you taught them so far?' he enquired.

The leader showed him a scruffy manual opened at the appropriate section of their course.

'I've been reading this bit out to the boys, so I think they should know it all by now.'

Mike had been a Boy Scout in his own formative years and thought that a practical emphasis could be more interesting than a simple reading of the material. Anyway, it was another opportunity to connect with the locals and cross-fertilise each other's ways of learning and doing.

'Maybe if I show them how to make slings, do bandaging and things like that, the boys could learn some useful skills,' he suggested tactfully.

'That'd be good. How many weeks do you need?' the leader asked with growing interest.

'Say four weeks I think, to get through these topics. Where do you meet?'

'The Catholic Church hall on Saturdays at two.'

'Sure,' Mike replied, 'I can bring some bandages and other gear from the hospital with me.'

The hall was a dilapidated venue with a rickety array of chairs and trestle tables and a dusty sink in one corner. About twenty boys attended and Mike led them through techniques for resuscitation, slings and splints for imaginary fractures, treating envenomations, and so forth. They practised their skills on each other amid a buzz of excited chatter after Mike demonstrated on volunteer patients. Most of the boys passed their exam with flying colours during the concluding session and he praised them for their excellent results.

The leader took Mike aside at the end of the last lesson. 'Mr Dr Browne, can you come back next week with your family? We want to say Thank you for your help.'

'Of course,' Mike smiled.

True to form, the boys' families hosted a small *kaikai* that all four of us attended and I brought some cakes along to share. The scouts demonstrated their new skills by applying various dressings and slings to our kids and one another. Mike also donated a First Aid kit of spare bits and pieces that he had scrounged from the hospital dispensary. He concluded his temporary leadership position by advising them to take the kit on their camps and scouting functions in the future, and gave a short speech on the imperative to always 'Be Prepared.'

Soon afterwards two challenging deliveries occurred in rapid succession involving 'grand multiparas': women who'd had five or more previous pregnancies. The first mama gave birth to a chubby ten-pound boy, who began life with eight older sisters. It seemed his parents had doggedly pursued their dream of having a male heir and their persistence was finally rewarded. His stocky dimensions suggested the possibility that his mama may have had gestational diabetes, so Mike arranged for her blood sugars to be checked postnatally. But the report revealed the usual default level of 6.3mmol/l, since the lab technician was probably drunk again. Consequently, the question (as did so many others during our islander posting) remained unresolved.

The other grand multipara was clearly made of stern stuff as well, as she fronted up for her thirteenth delivery. Mike was dismayed to discover that her baby had wriggled into a face presentation, meaning that instead of his head being flexed (chin on chest), his neck was extended backwards and his face looking outwards. This presentation made the delivery much more dangerous due to the risk of obstruction. To add to these difficulties, the mama's uterus was lax after so many previous deliveries and her contractions were irregular and weak. Mike had to use forceps to rotate the baby's head into a more favourable occipital position, before starting a Syntocinon infusion to get things moving along more efficiently. After many tedious hours, the baby and mama finally got their acts together and the infant put in his belated appearance.

Once again, when Mike arrived home, I had to listen carefully and give consoling grunts during his descriptions of these latest rollercoaster deliveries. Our extensive debriefs were essential for preserving his tenuous grasp on sanity after so many vivid and recurring labour-ward nightmares.

A measles outbreak presented further complexities at this time, since routine inoculations with Measles/Mumps/Rubella vaccine were sometimes missed by the locals. We saw a flurry of youngsters with the typical high fevers, watery eyes, snuffly noses and widespread spotty rashes. Pua led the nurses in a catch-up program of immunisations of the local children to try to limit the spread of the disease.

Several kids became seriously ill with measles pneumonia and required oxygen and intravenous antibiotics to assist in their recovery. Another girl developed measles encephalitis, a potentially lethal complication of this cruel viral illness. Raging fevers and wild convulsions wracked her young body, and led to weakness and serious weight loss.

We were greatly relieved when she eventually began to recover. In the end, she showed no long-term evidence of brain damage or other impairments and we discharged her back home after a lengthy hospital stay.

~

Outpatients had been fairly quiet one morning, when a couple carried in their one-year-old son, Arno. The baby had been vomiting and feverish on and off for about a week, but paralysing *akama* had hindered his parents from bringing him to the hospital earlier. We had found that some Māori, particularly those who had more difficulty with speaking English, shared the belief that they would be censured for having a sick child. It was an attitude that we found both puzzling and frustrating, as we didn't know how to counter it, and the language difficulties only made it more difficult to address.

'Come this way,' I said, leading them into the clinic room where I soon detected the rigidity of Arno's neck and the irritable jerky muscle tone of his limbs. I felt dismayed at the possible serious diagnoses that these features implied.

'I'll need to do a lumbar puncture,' I said soberly, 'I think he may have an infection in his brain called meningitis or encephalitis.'

They looked at me with horror – the words were confusing but full of fearful connotations. Kata helped to translate, as well as describing the procedure that I needed to do. We positioned Arno on his side with his legs curled into a foetal position: it opened up his intervertebral spaces so that I could slide in a needle and drain out some CSF. His cerebrospinal pressures were high and the clear fluid sent to the lab confirmed a viral encephalitis.

'Baby Arno has a serious brain infection,' I explained to his parents later that day, with Kata interpreting for me again; 'It doesn't usually get better with antibiotics, but I will give them anyway, just to try everything we can.'

As the nurse finished talking to the parents, abject fear was written all over their faces and I was moved by their distress.

'I'll also give him some other medicine called steroids to try to decrease the pressure inside his head. I hope that all these things will make a difference.'

But the tears gathering in my eyes betrayed my sense that this illness was not going to get better anytime soon.

The following day, Father Luke came to the hospital to baptise Arno: the baby's family and ours were all present. We crowded around the small cot, a huddle of grief that fumbled for courage in the face of so much uncertainty. Luke tenderly touched Arno's brow with water and oil – incanting ancient words of blessing and life. But any sense of hope continued to stubbornly recede.

I spoke to his parents afterwards. 'Arno needs to go to Raro tomorrow. He's not getting better and they may want to send him to New Zealand for further treatment.'

The parents nodded with silent resignation and went home to prepare for the trip. Mike went with them and the baby on the next day's flight to Raro Hospital, where Arno was treated for several days. When he failed to improve there, he was sent on to Greenlane Hospital in Auckland for months of care and rehabilitation, but all to no avail. Little Arno eventually returned to the island with irreversible brain damage and blindness. Worst of all, his prognosis remained very poor: he was unlikely to survive beyond childhood and his quality of life was pitiable indeed.

Like his parents, we also carried the weight of impotence and grief when patients failed to improve. These kinds of circumstances led to profound physical and emotional strains on both Mike and me, made worse by the frequent and unpredictable on-call demands. Many days melted into one another, in a blur of mind-numbing responsibility and exhaustion, and over these months, it became gradually harder to recover our drive and enthusiasm with the unrelenting challenges that we had to face.

Rather ironically, Mike received a letter about this time from the Royal Australian College of General Practitioners stating that, having submitted a log of patients he'd seen on Aitutaki thus far, he had now achieved a 'Certificate of Satisfactory Completion of Training.' This meant that he was now considered 'competent to work as an unsupervised practitioner in general primary care settings.'

This document was an extraordinarily trite understatement of the level of medical care that we'd been providing, mostly alone and without backup for the past twenty months. Our island medical caseloads and the absence of support services far exceeded anything that the average Australian GP would be required to handle, let alone those, like us, who were still progressing through their Family Medicine Program, and were supposedly still under the supervision of senior doctors.

It was gratifying to know that he was now officially 'allowed' to do the work that he'd already been doing for so long. Somehow though, I don't think that framing this certificate and putting it on the wall in Outpatients would have made the slightest difference to the islanders that we treated. They showed no reluctance in seeking out our care at all hours of the day and night, regardless of whether or not we possessed any official documentation to prove that we were appropriately qualified. They brought their manifold problems to us – we did our best – and ultimately, that seemed to be all that they desired.

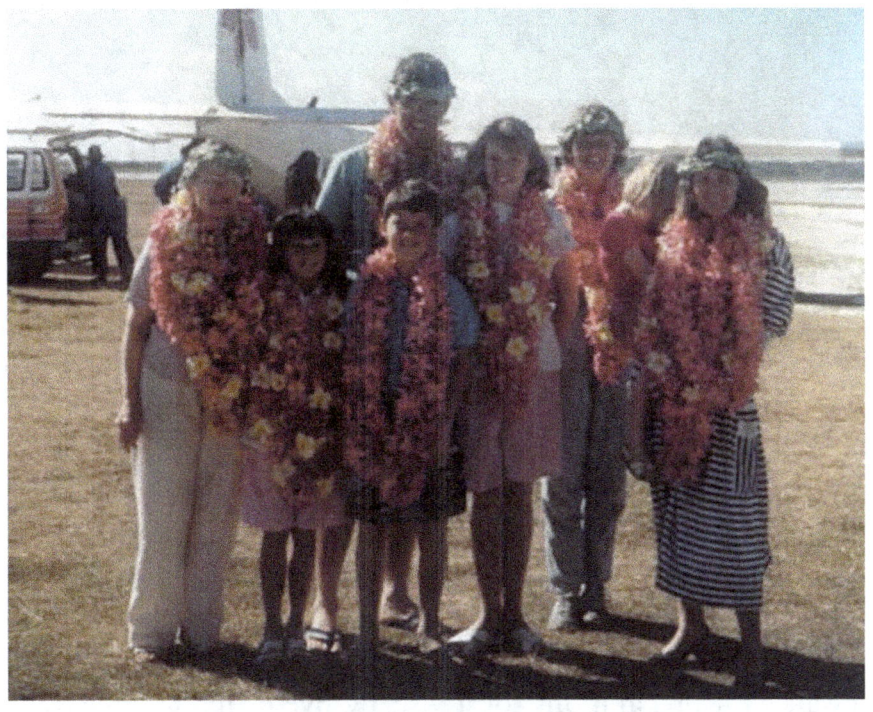

**Our visitors arrive!
Back row L>R: Philip Jones, Megan Hawkins.
Front row: Marguerite Cole, Sarah, Ben, Heidi, Marguerite Jones holding Bronwyn.**

30 – Visitors (Part III)
Theirs and Ours

In August 1989, it was time to bid farewell to our good friends Sam and Rachel – a sad day indeed. Their time on the island had gone far too quickly, and we knew we would miss their companionship and practical support enormously.

Meanwhile, we became caught up in assisting our friend Ewan with preparations for a visit by five of his UK relatives, who planned to stay with his family for several months. Since they hadn't been to Aitutaki for over ten years, they hadn't met Ewan's wife Kara or his daughters, Jane and Tina. It was a significant occasion for the whole household and Ewan was understandably anxious that all went well. We expressed our willingness to help in whatever way we could – and this entailed numerous jobs over the next few weeks.

Coincidentally, we had arranged to have a week of annual leave ourselves at this time, and had moved into the cottage at

Silcock's beach in an attempt to outwit the patients who came to the kitchen door at our place, whether we were technically 'on call' or not. We figured it might take them at least a few days to track us down, so it was worth a try anyway. As well as the change of scene, we had hoped we would also have a much-needed change of pace. But as it happened, our working life was simply replaced by the many tasks we did with our friends.

A few weeks earlier, Ewan had dropped over to our place one evening.

'Hey Mike, I was wondering if you know how to build a flush toilet?' he began.

I looked at Mike with a mixture of humour and amazement – it seemed there was no limit to the breadth of holistic skills that were expected of us on this tiny island.

Mike grinned. 'Mm, well I've never put one in before, but I'm happy to give it a go.'

'Yeah well I thought my family might not be too keen to use the long-drop in our backyard,' Ewan said, 'So if we could make an inside toilet, they wouldn't need to, huh?'

'Good thinking. Have you got any plans?'

'Well a plumber friend of mine has found me a spare toilet bowl. He's going away for a month so he can't help, but he was telling me how to put it in: it sounds pretty easy.'

He sounded confident, although I must admit, I had my doubts.

Shortly afterwards, when our leave began, Mike turned up to assist. A junk room adjacent to the back of Ewan's house had been ear-marked for this project and the two friends set to work. At one stage, Mike looked up from the depths of the septic pit he was digging to see Rhiannon with Jane picking flowers from the uppermost branches of a huge old *tipani* tree.

'Hi Dad,' Rhiannon said, leaning forward to see him better.

'Hi darl.' A sudden swoop of vertigo swirled around him as he imagined her falling from a great height and sustaining all kinds of serious injuries in the process.

'Be careful there, huh?' He realised how lame it sounded, in view of her risky location. But then again, she seemed to think that her parents were unnecessarily over-protective and that we should let her be more adventurous – so perhaps she was right.

She brushed off his anxiety with a nod: 'Sure.'

Mike turned back to the septic pit to avoid looking at her perilous position any longer.

Meanwhile, I assisted Kara with other tasks such as moving bags of cement and oil drums out of the kitchen, wiping down cupboards and sewing colourful curtains and cushion covers with a borrowed sewing machine.

Two-year-old Thomas played with Tina and went on occasional outings with the family. He was keen to re-enact for me his trip to the shops while standing on the steps of Kara's motor scooter: 'No bread at bakery – never mind – hold on tight to Kara's dress – don't let go – *careful* Thomas!'

Once again, I was glad that I hadn't been watching this venture. Our kids enjoyed the novelty of hanging out with Ewan's household and seemed to find their place much more interesting than ours. Thomas learned to chew gum while he was there – even managing to keep it in his mouth for seven hours straight whilst eating cold canned spaghetti and bowls of ice-cream – it was quite an impressive feat, really.

After three days of construction, the two men had completed a hand-dug septic tank and overflow, lined it with concrete, filled it with rubble, and cemented both the cover and the floor of the room. The toilet itself was then installed to connect with the ingoing and outgoing plumbing, an electric light attached to the ceiling, a packet of Blue Loo sprinkled into the bowl, a picture calendar affixed to the wall and a toilet-roll holder fashioned from a wire coat-hanger screwed to the wall. It was an epic piece of creativity by the enthusiastic amateurs. Thomas was invited to christen the device to ensure that it operated properly, and he fulfilled his role admirably. Thankfully, so did the loo.

After this success, Mike was tasked with butchering the fatted pig, one that he had previously castrated, then cutting it up and wrapping it in banana leaves for the *umukai*. While others made potato salad and *pok'e*, and prepared tubs of taro and *kumara* ready for the *umu*, I baked a dozen cakes. The night before the guests arrived, we helped to make a mountain of *eis* with the extended islander family. It was fun to be part of the welcoming party when the family alighted from their plane the following day, and to join in the numerous *kaikais* over the next few weeks.

All in all, it was a special time. Ewan had been such a good friend to us that it was gratifying to repay some of his kindness by supporting them in this valuable season of re-connection with his wider family.

~

After completing some finishing touches to the welcome cakes that I'd made, gathering up a box of *eis*, and chivvying the kids out of their morning distractions, I drove them to the large house that I had booked for my extended family to use during their two-week visit. A final sweep and the place looked ready, as Rhiannon placed a bright hibiscus in a cup in the middle of the table.

Suddenly it was ten o'clock – time to be at the airport.

In my belated dash in the car, I swerved on the narrow road and clipped a few somnolent chooks – possibly with lethal consequences. But there was no time to pause and check out the damage in our haste to meet our relatives.

Just as we arrived, the plane taxied to a halt on the runway, and the kids and I tumbled out of the car and watched as the passengers alighted. The plane gradually emptied, but with no sign of the eight people that we most wanted to see. While this happened fairly often, it was especially upsetting today, when we had looked forward so much to seeing our extended family. I went to the Cook Island Air counter with the kids, who were cross and dispirited by now.

'Any ideas when they're likely to come?'

'No, Mrs Dr Browne,' the local replied. 'Try again at 1 p.m. – maybe they'll be arriving on the next plane by then.'

I sighed. There never seemed to be any explanation for the erratic and unannounced changes to flight schedules and passenger records. The *eis* that we'd made the night before would be starting to brown and shrivel by that time I thought, even if we placed them in the shade.

I contrived a cheerful smile as I turned to the kids: 'Let's go home for morning tea and we'll come back at lunchtime.'

I checked for signs of chicken corpses on the way back, without mentioning this to the kids – they didn't need something else to fret about. But thankfully none were in evidence: maybe I hadn't subjected any to mortal injuries after all, or perhaps the pragmatic locals were already preparing them for dinner. Either way, there didn't seem to be anyone looking for an apology or payment – so I drove home at a sedate pace, with careful attention to the road conditions this time.

When we returned for the next flight, my mother, an old friend called Megan, and my sister's family all appeared, tired but thankful to have arrived at last. They enjoyed the slightly spent *eis* as we warmly welcomed them and I ferried them back to our place for a late lunch. Despite the noise and crowding, it was a lot of fun.

When Mike arrived home, we shared with them the exciting news that we were now expecting our third child, who was due to arrive about 18th May, 1990. We didn't tell our kids much about my pregnancy at this stage, as we knew that the wait for their new sibling would seem inordinately long for them otherwise.

At one stage, we had wondered about having a baby while we were still in the Cooks, as the Vandermoezels and our Mauke friends had done before us. But feeling the weight of work-stress and isolation for much of the time already, we had decided to start number three on the island and finish in Australia instead. Ultimately, we knew that we'd prefer to have our family and friends closer to hand for this next chapter in the tale of our family life.

Once again, while having visitors, we took the opportunity to do more touristy things than usual: *motu* trips, Island Night, meals out, fishing and reef explorations, and going to the church services that had the best music. Thomas enjoyed participating in hymns, although he heartily sang his favourite song: 'Happy Birthday to Me' with all of them. The main downside was that he didn't stop when the congregation sat down, much to the amusement of the locals, so he had to be whisked outside until he finally ground to a halt. By then, he was more interested in the goats outside than the service itself, so he didn't want to go back until the next hymn began. All this led to a rather disrupted church experience for whoever was on parental duties that day.

The long hot church services that we often attended were usually conducted entirely in Māori. Since they were of little interest to our children, we had commenced a small Sunday School at our place for our kids, and the others who joined us included some of our *papa'a* neighbours, Jane and Tina, and the four cousins during their stay. The youngsters enjoyed the stories, songs and activities, with some helpful resources provided by my sister.

Our kids were keen to teach their relatives how to shred coconuts, squeeze out coconut milk, flavour home-made yoghurt with mashed fruit, and crack open *kaivi* to eat the inner almond-shaped seeds. They loved to share their own stories of island life too.

For the previous six months, Rhiannon had attended Preschool for five mornings each week from 8.00 till 10.00 a.m. It was hard for us to understand exactly what went on there, as her explanations ranged anywhere from the ordinary to the bizarre:

'We saw a rat in Preschool today' (that was fairly common).

Or, seeing her teacher ride past on her motorbike, she said: 'She really is a *dreadful* teacher. All she ever talks about is *monkeys* – it gets *so* boring.'

What was that supposed to mean, since obviously the island was devoid of these mammals?

Despite such assertions, however, she was rapidly becoming fluent in Māori and learning a vast vocabulary of new words: counting to fifty, days of the week, months of the year, shapes, colours, and so on. She taught her cousins some of these words, along with islander dance steps, and all of the kids put on some group concerts for the adults' entertainment as well. Of course, being the youngest, Thomas tried to outdo the others by singing his favourite song at the top of his voice over and over again!

31 – Taxing Times

Those who volunteered through the Overseas Services Bureau (OSB) were employed directly by the government of their designated countries, so they were paid the equivalent salaries, and incurred the same expenses and taxes, as their local colleagues. Volunteers were also expected to live under equivalent housing and work conditions as their indigenous counterparts.

During our posting, Michael and I had a combined salary for one doctor working full time, and significant overtime, of $18,000 per year in New Zealand dollars (NZD). At the exchange rate at that time (1.30 NZD: 1.00 AUD), this was approximately $13,800 in Australian dollars (AUD) per year. Of this, 30% was deducted automatically for Cook Islands tax and a further 15% for house rental, leaving us with $7,600 AUD on which to live for each year on the island. This equated to $146 AUD nett per week for our total workload, or about $2 per hour.

In mid-1989, we received an unexpected income tax return of $1000 AUD from the Australian Tax Office, the ATO. Their enclosed letter explained that we were owed the refund because we had overpaid our Australian tax – a surprising but welcome adjustment, as our financial circumstances during our OSB contract were modest, to say the least.

Some weeks later however, having banked the refund cheque, we received a second letter from the ATO demanding that we repay $750 AUD immediately. *Maybe that's why they called it a 'return',* I thought!

It seemed that they had miscalculated our original refund. *If it seems too good to be true, it probably is too good to be true...*

The reason they gave for their faulty sums was that they'd had difficulty working out our 'residency status.'

At this stage, OSB had been in existence since 1963 and had celebrated its 25th anniversary in 1988. The organisation produced a report for each financial year, and the one for 1987-88 happened to feature Mike on the front cover, examining a small Māori baby alongside a local nurse at Aitutaki Hospital. From my biased perspective, it was the most interesting part of the entire document, of course!

This report stated that by mid-1988, two thousand volunteers had been sent through the programme to thirty-six developing countries. One would have expected therefore that, from their large number of previous cases, the ATO should have encountered and resolved the 'residency status' issue of volunteers by then. But evidently, this was not the case.

The personal cost of working in these roles was part of the contribution that we had all made to our host countries, but this was also magnified by other financial aspects of volunteering. The report itself stated that 57% of OSB's budget at this time came from volunteers foregoing their usual salaries, long service leave, superannuation and other entitlements during their contract periods. This was a deliberate and pre-emptive choice that we had all made, so we didn't anticipate any particular acknowledgement for these sacrifices.

However, we weren't expecting to be targeted by our own taxation department either. Specifically, we were dismayed to discover that the ATO would exact additional taxes from us for whatever puny gains we had made while we were working as volunteers.

In our case, the only personal income that we had accrued in Australia during our posting was the rent on our Canberra house of $150 per week; it paid for our mortgage during our absence and totalled $7,800 AUD per year. This amount wouldn't even have qualified as taxable income by usual Australian rates at the time.

However, in its wisdom, the ATO chose to apply a formula known as 'grossing up' to calculate our tax liabilities. This entailed adding together our Australian rental income with our gross Cook Islands income, ignoring the fact that we had already paid 30% tax to the Cook Islands' government, and then charging us tax at the usual Australian tax rate. Consequently, in addition to the $750 that they had demanded back from us during our posting, additional levies were exacted from us after we arrived home. This felt very unfair.

Apparently, the original 'grossing up' arrangement had been designed by the ATO to extract tax from Australian businesses who had made or banked their profits overseas in order to evade their local pecuniary obligations. We heard from OSB that they had repeatedly contacted the ATO on behalf of all volunteers who were affected by this policy, in order to try to negotiate a waiver for lowly-paid aid-workers. However, it seemed that OSB's petitions had fallen on deaf ears. We hope that these arrangements have been amended since that time.

Several months after returning to Australia, along with

numerous other volunteers, we received letters and certificates at an OSB ceremony in Canberra to thank us for the 'tremendous contribution' we had made to developing nations through our volunteer labours. Politicians were lining up at the event to have their photos taken with us, all trying to look as caring, sensitive and committed as we probably did at our first briefing. We couldn't help but feel that the political environment that we'd experienced in the Cooks was simply a microcosm of the version that existed in many western countries, including our own. Spin, image and being seen in the right places alongside the most politically correct citizens is the bread-and-butter of political success everywhere, it seemed.

Consequently, we felt even more insulted when several weeks after this event, we received another letter from the ATO, this time demanding that we pay them an additional $500 AUD because of a further adjustment in their formula for determining our tax liabilities. We didn't even have that amount of spare cash at the time, since it equalled nearly a month's income for us on Aitutaki, and we hadn't been able to save much on our local salary. We had to borrow the sum from relatives until we could pay them back, once we began working in Australia again.

This taxation demand was just one of several ironic double messages that we received from our own political system, both during and after our volunteer posting, as 'ambassadors' for our country. It was a peculiar and paradoxical way for those in government to hand out their certificates, line up to have their photos taken with us, and proclaim with shrewd sincerity:

'Welcome home folks!'

32 – Herculean Heroics

In October '89, we faced yet another escalation in the numbers and complexity of our medical caseload. The burden of these challenging presentations, as well as our shrinking social supports, drained our resilience considerably. Although we were excited about my third pregnancy, I was drained by fatigue and nausea, and found it hard to continue to work at my previous pace. I discovered that unexpected things could provoke my symptoms – even seeing a fish in our freezer was enough to trigger quite a nasty bout of retching.

Around this time, a New Zealand army contingent had arrived on the island and camped in scrubland near the airport. They practised bush skills, engaged in military manoeuvres and repaired various dilapidated buildings during their stay. One morning, an army doctor came up to Outpatients with a private, who nursed a bleeding hand wrapped in bandages.

'Hi there, I'm Captain Rory Weston.' The Kiwi doctor shook Mike's hand. 'Young Martin here was helping to demolish an old fence and forgot to wear his protective gloves. He's managed to prang his hand with some big splinters of wood.'

'Ok, let's have a look then,' Mike said as he took off the bandages and examined the man's bleeding limb. 'Mm, I think we'll need to take him to theatre and debride it under a nerve block.'

The captain nodded. 'Yeah, that's what I thought too. But it was a bit more than we could manage with our basic resources.'

They helped the young man onto the theatre bed, and one of the nurses cleaned him up with warm water and antiseptic. His hand was an ugly mass of wood and blood, and he flinched with pain as the fluids doused his raw flesh.

Mike drew up a syringe of local anaesthetic and inserted a brachial nerve block to numb his arm. Once the medication kicked in, the distressed private dropped into a more relaxed state and became rather drowsy. With Weston's assistance, Mike debrided the wound, removing large splinters of rotten wood, then wrapped clean dressings around his hand. He finished off with intramuscular Penicillin and checked that Martin's tetanus status was up to date.

The Kiwi doctor was grateful. 'Good job! That would've been quite tricky for me to do in our bush tent.'

'Well, I'm not sure that our facilities are much better than yours,' Mike smiled and Weston nodded as he looked around the theatre.

'Yeah, I see what you mean. Hey, what should we do about aftercare?' the Kiwi asked.

'It might be best to keep him here overnight to make sure there's no sign of infection, I think.' Mike scrubbed off his hands and began to tidy up the surgical gear. Martin appeared to be quite pale and groggy, so the captain agreed with this suggestion.

Before heading back to their temporary base, Weston confirmed that he'd be back the following day to collect the young private. He also added that the army unit would be happy to donate any of their residual medical supplies when they left the island, and Mike gladly accepted his offer. Any contributions to our dwindling dispensary supplies were always welcome.

A few nights later, having completed another long delivery on his 'weekend off,' Mike noticed the operating theatre lights were on as he wearily trudged through the hospital. It was an unusual event for a Saturday at midnight. As a sense of foreboding settled over him, he took a deep breath, trying to find some sparse reserves of energy and focus before going to investigate.

He found Dr Rua bending over the theatre bed where a semi-comatose man was lying. The young islander was sweating profusely and looked a disturbing shade of blue-grey; his heavy breathing and painful groans as he clutched his belly all indicated something seriously wrong. Dr Rua looked up hopefully as Mike entered the room.

'Hi there, what's happened to him?' Mike asked.

'Kopu's epileptic. His family found him tonight under a coconut tree, so I think he must've had a fit and fallen down.'

'Gosh – do you want some help?' Mike knew that he'd have wanted whatever assistance was on offer in his colleague's place.

Ragged with worry and fatigue, Dr Rua nodded keenly: 'Yeah, that'd be good.'

Mike checked over the patient's limbs and found them mercifully intact, but as he felt Kopu's belly, he noticed that it was as hard as a board and the young man cried out in pain. Mike suspected that he'd probably suffered intra-abdominal injuries and blood loss during his fall.

'We'd better put in some large-bore cannulae – he's going to need as much fluid as we can get into him, I think.' Mike stretched his back as he focused on a possible plan.

A young nurse stood by, anxious and uncertain in the ominous atmosphere of the theatre.

Mike turned to her and said: 'Could you ring for the technician? We're going to need blood donors as soon as possible, thanks.' She disappeared without a word.

The two doctors worked together to insert plasma, as well as a urinary catheter, naso-gastric tube, and oxygen mask. The technician was summoned and, being surprisingly sober on this occasion, got down to the job of cross-matching blood and rounding up locals for the usual donor-to-patient transfusions.

At this point, Mike could see that Dr Rua was limp with exhaustion and said: 'There's no need for both of us to be here now. How about you go home and get some rest?'

The older man nodded gratefully and left.

It was about 3 a.m. on Sunday by now, with no domestic flights available until 9 a.m. Monday. Although his body ached with weariness, Mike's thoughts ricocheted along fruitless tracks with no apparent solution around how to get Kopu to Raro for emergency surgery. The transfusions were running and would continue for many hours yet. Eventually, with nothing more that could be done at this time of day, Mike decided to head home as well, to try to get some sleep.

Several hours later, Mike and I talked and prayed through this tangled quandary: Kopu clearly needed an urgent laparotomy to repair his internal injuries before he bled to death, but we had no idea of how to get him to Raro Hospital in time. A knot of anxiety tightened inside us both as Mike returned to the hospital about 7 a.m.

He decided to assess Kopu further by doing a peritoneal lavage – a technique that required the use of a very large-bore cannula: a black dwell-cath with the same diameter as a drinking straw. This procedure involved running a litre of sterile saline into the patient's abdomen via the dwell-cath, then placing the giving set on the floor to allow the fluid to drain back into the plastic tubing. The old-fashioned rule of thumb went something like this: if you could still read newsprint through the fluid in the tubing, the internal bleeding was mild to moderate. If the newsprint was illegible, due to the density of blood in the aspirate, the bleeding was severe. On this occasion, the fluid was deeply blood-stained, indicating that Kopu's haemorrhaging was emphatically life-threatening.

It was time to investigate extraordinary measures to get this young man to surgery as soon as possible.

Mike started with some phone calls – firstly to the Director General of Health in Rarotonga (who was indignant at being roused so early on a Sunday morning), then the airport desk at Cook Island Air in Rarotonga, and lastly the Aitutaki airport manager. In the end, it was the latter who proved to be the most useful, as he pointed out that, quite remarkably, there was a New Zealand Airforce C130 Hercules currently parked on the Aitutaki runway.

Apparently, the reason for this very rare occurrence was that the plane was being used for a United Nations seed-farming project. Trochus shells were being harvested from the Aitutaki lagoon and placed in sacks ready for the aircraft to deposit them into the waters off Tuvalu and Tokelau, thereby providing an alternative income source for these small Pacific islands. Thankfully however, the Hercules crew were observing the obligatory day of rest according to islander custom, so the plane was stationary on the airport tarmac at the time.

At last, Mike sensed a glimmer of hope for Kopu and eagerly asked the telephonist to put him through to the Hercules air force crew.

'Hello, this is Dr Mike Browne from Aitutaki Hospital,' he

began when the phone was answered.

'Hello, Major Benton here,' the Kiwi responded.

'Good. I understand you're on the island with your Hercules and wondered if we could ask for your help,' Mike continued.

An awkward pause followed. 'Mm, well I think you've got the wrong team then, doctor,' came the distinctly gruff reply; 'I'm in a tent with the *army* deployment at present. We're in the bush campsite near the airport.'

'Oh,' Mike responded with some initial confusion, and then he remembered his recent contact with the unit; 'Yes, of course. So, would you happen to know where I can find the Hercules crew then?'

There was an icy note in the major's voice as he hissed each syllable in reply: 'I believe they're located in the Akitua Resort Hotel.'

'Ah.' Mike suddenly understood the major's frigid tone. The marked discrepancy in status and accommodation standards between the two Kiwi military groups was obviously a sore point already, and it would be imprudent to labour the point any further.

'Uh-huh – well, thank you so much for your assistance, Major,' he added politely, and heard a loud 'Humph' on the line before hanging up.

Trying the telephonist again, he asked to be put through to the resort. After more stops and starts and crackling on the line, he was finally connected to the air crew officer.

'Hello, it's Dr Mike Browne from Aitutaki Hospital,' he began again, 'Can you hear me ok?'

The officer spoke briskly: 'Roger, you're all ahead straight five, sir.'

'Oh, er – right. Who am I speaking to?'

'It's Flight-Lieutenant Haynes here, sir, of the Royal New

Zealand Airforce.'

'Good. I was wondering if we could borrow your plane?'

'Really?' The Kiwi responded more cautiously.

'Yes, well we've got a serious medical emergency here,' Mike explained, 'A young man's fallen from a coconut tree and has life-threatening internal injuries. We need to get him to Rarotonga Hospital for abdominal surgery as soon as possible, or he's likely to bleed to death within the next six to twelve hours.'

'Right – well in that case, I'm authorised to make that decision.' The Flight-Lieutenant sensed that he was now on more certain territory. 'That's no problem at all. We can be airborne in ninety minutes at your service, sir.'

A surge of euphoria finally broke through the deep gloom of the past long hours and Mike responded with a rush of elation in his voice: 'Thank you so much, Flight-Lieutenant – that is *great!*' he said, almost sobbing with relief.

Once he'd recovered his equilibrium, he rang Raro Hospital to alert them of the proposed transfer so that they could prepare for immediate surgery on their arrival.

Somewhat unexpectedly, the Director General of Health rang Mike back an hour later to say that, following discussions with the New Zealand High Commissioner and the Minister for Defence, he had ascertained that there was a New Zealand Airforce Hercules on Aitutaki that was available for our use. It took Mike some time to convince the Director that he, a mere doctor, had circumvented official channels, and the pilot was already preparing for departure at 1100 hours. The Director was initially brusque at being surplus to requirements, but soon expressed his pleasure that the problem had been resolved to everyone's satisfaction.

By now it was 9.10 a.m. and there was a tight schedule ahead, as it takes some time to prepare a patient for transfer and he was still being transfused. The Hercules also needed to be readied for the flight and Mike had been informed of a mechanical problem with the plane that may have meant their transfer and return flight could be delayed.

Along with these issues, there was another small complication: Mike had been engaged to preach the sermon at the Vaipae Presbyterian Church that morning.

So his crowded timetable went something like this:

9.15 – 9.35 a.m. – Ate, showered, shaved and packed a small bag for a possible overnight stay in Raro.

9.35 – 9.55 a.m. – Checked the patient and oxygen cylinder, replaced the naso-gastric tube, re-inserted an IV cannula to complete the third transfusion and packed an emergency medical transfer kit.

9.55 – 10.15 a.m. – I drove all four of us to the Vaipae church and Mike delivered his sermon at the beginning of the service instead of at the end.

10.15 – 10.50 a.m. – I drove us back to the hospital where we re-checked Kopu and loaded him and the necessary equipment into the ambulance. The driver then took them all to the airport and I followed with the kids in our car.

10.55 – 11.00 a.m. – The four of us were introduced to the eight Royal New Zealand Airforce Hercules crew.

As so often happens in these unusual circumstances, there were further last-minute problems: the technical hitch with the aircraft, which may have meant they'd be unable to return to Aitutaki on the same day, had also delayed their departure until 12.15 p.m. The mechanics finally resolved the issue, the patient and medical gear were loaded on board, and the Hercules was ready for take-off.

The crew was very merry despite this interruption to their rest day – the idea of being heroes appealed to them considerably, it seemed. We were both still thrilled with the extraordinary provision of the plane, and the kids and I waved them all off enthusiastically.

Mike spent the flight kneeling on the plane's steel floor next to Kopu's stretcher, and held the oxygen mask in position in a very hot and noisy part of the aircraft. The unconscious patient was strapped in and oblivious to all the commotion occurring around him. The flight lasted thirty minutes, half the time taken by a commercial flight, and they were met on arrival by an ambulance that whisked patient and doctor to Raro Hospital, where the operating theatre staff was remarkably well prepared for the emergency surgery.

Mike was expecting to assist in the procedure and was scrubbing up to do so, when a call came through to the hospital from the Hercules Flight-Lieutenant. He informed Mike that the plane's mechanical fault had now been fully repaired, the crew was ready for the return flight and he was welcome to join them if he wished. He had already seized the opportunity of stuffing his backpack with various supplies that we needed from the hospital dispensary, so bidding his Raro colleagues farewell, he grabbed his gear and jumped into a spare ambulance to return to the airport as soon as possible.

Flight-Lieutenant Haynes invited Mike to sit behind the flight deck near the pilot and they witnessed amazing views throughout the journey back. The crew was in high spirits since they could resume their resort stay earlier than expected, and they all munched on mini-pizzas from the plane's galley for a late lunch. Mike soon regretted his snack though, due to the overpowering nausea created by the turbulent flight.

The pilot flew a bone-bending double-fly past Aitutaki at 250 feet, pitched at about thirty degrees, where the G-forces were so powerful that Mike could barely lift his arms. All of his photos of this trip are distinctly side-on!

Hearing the thunderous low-flying aircraft overhead, I soon realised that the Hercules was returning the same day after all, so the kids and I dived into the car and drove back to the airport where the plane was just coming in to land. After Mike briefed me on Kopu's successful transfer, the crew showed us around their impressive craft and allowed the kids to sit at the flight desk and 'fly' the plane. Their eyes were like saucers between the large headphones, and Thomas even agreed that this experience superseded the thrill of driving 'hooge 'normous diggers.'

We gave the crew our warm thanks for their remarkable assistance. It was truly miraculous that, on the one occasion during our posting when we desperately needed to get someone off the island for immediate life-saving interventions, a plane and crew were available to do so. Our joy and gratitude knew no bounds!

We found out subsequently that Kopu had ruptured his liver, right kidney and duodenum, all of which were successfully repaired by the Raro surgical team. He returned to Aitutaki four weeks later and made a slow but complete recovery.

We later wrote a letter of thanks to the New Zealand Ministry of Defence, commending the cheerful professionalism of the Hercules crew and their timely assistance. Without a doubt, the bold requests, emergency interventions and good-hearted collaboration of everyone involved had saved this young man's life, and this episode remains a very positive landmark in our reflections of the many highs and lows of our tropical sojourn.

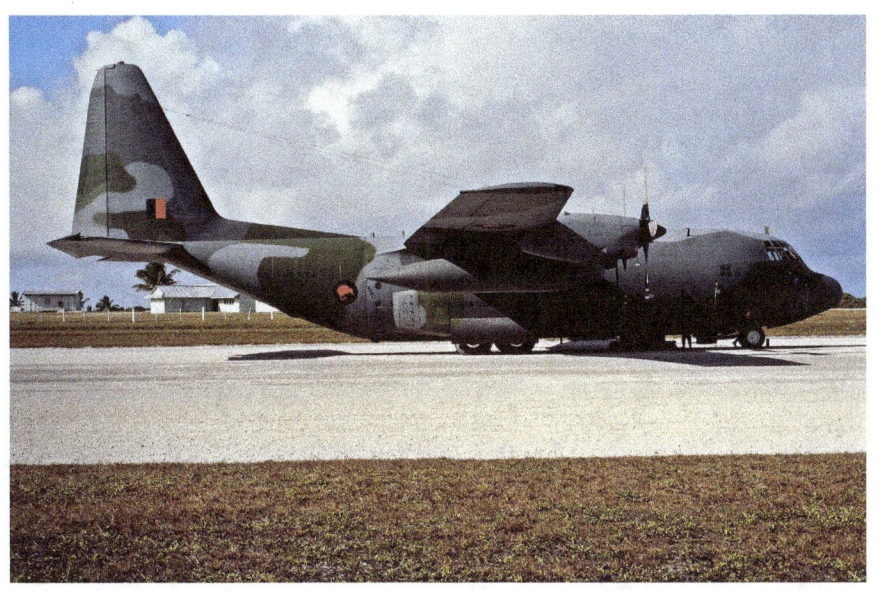

Royal New Zealand Airforce C130 Hercules on Aitutaki runway.

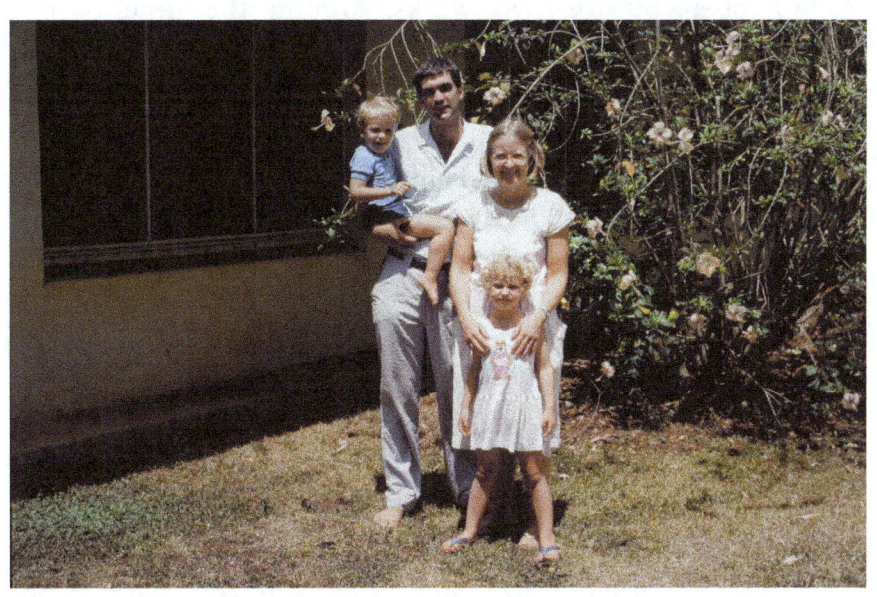

**Our family outside our house – mid-October 1989.
Photo taken by Felix.**

33 – Final Days

Our last visitor to Aitutaki arrived to stay with us in mid-October '89 for two weeks, around the time of our Hercules adventure. We had originally met Felix in Switzerland on a five-month European trip that we had made in 1984, and we'd stayed in touch with him and his parents ever since. Having an engineering background, Felix impressed our kids with his creative Duplo constructions, and he explored the island with the careful attention and detailed record-keeping that characterise the Swiss.

We prepared morning tea as he returned from a long walk and sat down at the dining-room table.

'So, what are your plans for going back to Australia?' Felix asked.

'Well, we haven't used much of our annual leave during our posting, so we thought we'd use some of that to head home early – probably about late November,' Mike said as he handed out mugs of hot tea and I cut up a loaf of home-made banana bread.

'Do you feel like you were well-prepared for your time here?'

Felix continued as he picked up a slice.

'Well, we were fortunate to be able to write back and forth to the Vandermoezels, the family that was here before us,' Mike replied; 'They gave us some helpful advice that made a big difference to us. We wouldn't have thought of bringing our car, for instance, if they hadn't suggested it.'

'Mm, that *is* a surprising thing for them to recommend,' our friend agreed.

Mike sipped his tea. 'It was useful to get their feedback and we *are* very glad that we've had the car here – it's been great. But of course, hearing about this place was very different from living here – no one can really prepare you for that – you've just got to find out for yourself.'

'Yes, I'm sure,' Felix replied, topping up his mug from the teapot; 'I guess you'll have lots to get done before leaving the island. What will you do with all the household things – you wouldn't want to take them with you, would you?'

'No that's for sure,' I agreed; 'We found out a few weeks ago that a Canadian couple with their two kids are coming to take over from us early next year. They'll need the same bits and pieces as us, so we've written to ask them if they want to buy our stuff from us, and we'll store it all for them, just as the Vandermoezels did for us.'

'That's a good idea – it works for you and for them,' Felix replied as the kids wandered in and began helping themselves to cake.

'Yes, it was certainly good for us to have so much useful gear when we first arrived,' I agreed.

'Once we tracked it all down!' Mike grinned as he explained that many of the items had gone AWOL. Our friend laughed appreciatively as Mike finished off with the anecdote about our thank-you gifts.

'Well, I can certainly see why the staff would enjoy your cooking,' he said, picking up another slice.

'I like cake,' Thomas said, as he crammed a large piece into his mouth.

'Are you going directly back to Australia?' Felix asked.

'No, we're going to see Sam and Rachel aren't we Mum?' Rhiannon said, discreetly taking another slice off the plate.

'That's right darling,' I replied, before turning back to Felix, 'They're a Kiwi couple that we met earlier this year when they came here for four months. We're hoping to spend a few days at their place on our stopover in Auckland, on the way back home.'

'I like Sam and Rachel,' Thomas added, with his mouth still full.

'Yes, we all do,' Mike said, 'They've been very special friends and we really miss them.'

I smiled at Mike and rose from the table: 'And I think it's time I cleared away the morning tea, before we all miss the banana bread too.'

I picked up the plate and headed for the kitchen.

~

A few days later, I came out of our bathroom with a horrible sense of dread churning within me. When Mike arrived home and saw my distress, he asked what was wrong.

I took him into our bedroom and shut the door as tears began to course down my face.

'I've had some bleeding,' I said, 'And I'm worried about what it might mean for the baby.'

We sat down together on the bed and he put his arm around my shoulders.

'Mm, that's not good. How many weeks are you now?'

'Nearly twelve weeks, so I'd thought I was past the most high-risk time,' I replied, wiping my face with a handkerchief.

'Have you had any pain?'

'No, thank goodness – that's one good sign at least.' I took a deep breath to try to settle my fears.

'Well, it's difficult since we don't have access to an ultrasound here, to see if the pregnancy is still viable. How do you feel about flying over to Raro to have one done there?'

I frowned and thought quietly for a few minutes. 'I've been wondering about that already this afternoon. I'd hate to have to do that by myself, especially if the news wasn't good – and if you were to come, we'd really need to take all of us, or else we'd need to explain the whole story to someone else. And anyway, Felix is here as well…'

'Mm, it would be awkward for him to mind our kids, or to be here without us – either way,' Mike added.

'Yes, exactly. Well, as you know, I had some bleeding with both of the other kids' pregnancies, so I keep hoping and praying that everything will settle down, as it did for them. Maybe it's just a small glitch that will soon get better,' I added, trying to sound more positive than I felt.

Mike nodded and we hugged each other, unsure of what else to say.

Unfortunately, however, the bleeding became a little heavier over the next few days, and I developed grumbling abdominal pain as well. I rested whenever I could, hoping that these things would soon resolve, but they seemed to persist regardless. The uncertainty and limited options weighed heavily on us and increased our angst considerably.

It was an intensely lonely and distressing time.

On Saturday, about a week later, we were all invited to afternoon tea by Margaret, a single *papa'a* woman who taught at the High School and had a seven-year-old son called Anton. She had heard that we'd be returning to Australia soon and was keen to acquire our home-made furniture when we left. I had felt a little better that day, so I decided to go along with the others, keen to have something else to focus on rather than my symptoms.

It was pleasant to be hosted at her place, but during the visit my bleeding suddenly intensified. I raced to the toilet and began to pass large clots with every recurring painful cramp and realised that I was haemorrhaging quite badly.

'We need to go,' I whispered to Mike with panicky urgency when I came back into the living room, 'It's getting really awful.'

I could no longer restrain the tears that flooded down my cheeks and fled from the house. Mike followed me out and we discussed what we needed to do next.

When he returned inside, Mike spoke quietly to Margaret: 'I'm sorry but Michele's not feeling at all well. Would you mind if Rhiannon stays to play with Anton for a while and I'll come and get her later?'

She agreed with a smile as she saw the two kids enjoying each other's company.

Mike drove Thomas, Felix and me back to our place and explained the situation to our friend. He was dismayed to hear of what we were going through, and offered to take care of Thomas while we both went up to the hospital. Mike rang Dr Rua to meet us there and we sat in mute distress in our consulting room until he arrived.

I was too upset to speak, so Mike explained: 'Michele's thirteen weeks pregnant, but it looks like she's having a miscarriage – she's haemorrhaging badly and her pain's really severe. Since there are no flights till Monday, I'm going to need to do a D&C myself.'

Dr Rua realised what a terrible predicament this was for both of us and simply nodded briefly.

'Do you want me to do the anaesthetic?' he asked quietly. We gratefully accepted his offer.

I was overwhelmed with sorrow for our baby, for Mike and for me. It was one of the most difficult things we'd ever had to face, both as doctors and as parents, and amplified our sense of isolation in every possible way. Not only was there the trauma of going through such a procedure so far from home, but Mike also had to carry the weight of being simultaneously doctor, spouse and parent in this situation – such a complex tangle of conflicting feelings and responsibilities. He was relieved when it was all over and he could drive me home for my post-op recovery.

We were glad that we hadn't told the kids much about our pregnancy in the first place, as they were both quite oblivious to what was happening. In his anxiety that I may have woken up before the end of the procedure, Dr Rua had given me twice the usual anaesthetic dose, so I was bed-bound for the next few days and had difficulty even walking from the bedroom to the bathroom.

Apart from that, the curette was successful in settling my heavy bleeding and pain. The procedure also confirmed that I'd had a blighted ovum (a non-viable pregnancy), so it could never have progressed to a normal outcome, either in Aitutaki or Australia. We were grateful that we didn't have to bear any sense of added guilt that we had intervened too soon: a small source of comfort in what was otherwise a uniformly bleak time.

Mike sent a telegram to the Director General of Health, stating that we needed to get home to Australia earlier than planned, due to my health issues, and to ensure that we all got the support and follow-up that we so desperately needed. Neither of us was able to manage the medical care of others when we could scarcely deal with our own. Shortly afterwards, when Felix left the island, we received official approval for us to leave Aitutaki on 6th November.

Coincidentally, the edge of a cyclone was passing to the north of the island at this time, causing wild weather and making radio-telephone contact with Raro virtually impossible. We were therefore unable to make plane bookings for our flights from the Cooks to Australia, so we had to hope and pray that our travel plans could be coordinated from the main island when we got there.

We planned to spend several days in Raro in a motel, to ensure that our flights to Australia were finalised and to close off our accounts with shops and banks. We also needed to contact the Stephens and our own families to notify them of our changed travel plans. Because of my poor health, we decided that we could only see our Kiwi friends for several hours during our stopover at Auckland airport, rather than stay with them at their home, as our highest priority was to get back to Australia as soon as possible, preferably by 10th November.

Our final days on Aitutaki remain a blur for both of us: for me due to blood loss, anaesthetic haze, and the ravages of grief; and for Mike with his own sense of loss, as well as balancing up his final work commitments while caring for us all. Our loneliness and heartache felt extreme for much of this time. Of course, we had the packing and children to attend to as well. The kids picked up on our low mood and would sometimes cry inconsolably for hours, which triggered my sadness yet again. We tried our best to reassure each other with hugs, reading books or playing low-key games to bring some distractions and lift our spirits, but these had only variable success.

One lighter memory we have of this time was that we recorded the kids on a cassette tape on our last night in our island home as they sang and chatted with us. Rhiannon bounced on the cane lounge as she reeled off numerous songs in Māori:

'One green bottle standing on the wall…
Twenty-two green bottles standing on the wall…
Forty-six green bottles standing on the wall…'

It did get a little tedious towards the end.

'I can make noises like the animals,' Thomas declared and followed up with accurate impersonations of all of the ones he knew. He answered some simple questions as well, and concluded his contribution with an amusing pun: 'I'm Thomas and I'm two – too much!'

Dr. Rua, who had always been a gracious colleague, waved aside his intention to retire (now for the third time) and modestly agreed to resume the mantle of 24/7 cover yet again, until the Canadian doctor arrived to share the load. As to what would happen with any obstetric cases that arose during these months, we presumed that he would have to deal with them himself, regardless of his preferences, just as he had had to do on previous occasions when he'd been obliged to work alone.

Our very ambivalent emotions at this time included a sense of guilt that we were abandoning our roles as doctors, and thereby putting the health of the Māori at risk. But we had to remind ourselves that this responsibility belonged to those in positions of governance. We had come and played our parts as diligently as possible, but now it was time for us to go and to pass on these tasks to others, who would have to take up the challenges that we could no longer bear.

As always, the hospital employees were very kind to us. They hosted a small farewell *kaikai* at the staffroom, and presented us with a beautiful blue *tivaevae* with matching cushions that the female staff had sewn by hand during the previous few months. We still treasure these gifts as tokens of the gratitude and esteem in which we held one another during our stay.

On the morning of our departure, a surreal sense settled over me as I walked around the house and garden for the last time. Each place held so many memories of all that we had experienced there: fear and peace, isolation and friendship, heartache and laughter, terror and relief…

The staff arrived on the ambulances with vast quantities of *eis* for us. They helped to load our suitcases into our car and the utes for our final trip across the island. When we arrived at the airport, we discovered many more familiar faces, both locals and *papa'as,* with a further abundance of *eis.* The kids were excited but fragile, and I found myself overcome by loss once again. Grief stubbornly simmered just below the surface of our lives.

We handed over the keys of the car to the guest-house owner Warren, who had purchased her from us several days earlier. It felt strange, having arrived with so much baggage in our trusty vehicle, to be departing now with just a suitcase and backpack each. Somehow it seemed symbolic though, that we were leaving a large part of ourselves behind on the island. Yet the smiles and *eis,* words and embraces, all told another tale too: that we would also carry much within us that was unique, crazy and precious, to inhabit our memories and way of life for many years to come.

Countless hugs were exchanged, beautiful hymns sung and prayers uttered, while the tears flowed freely, mingling together as our faces touched and dripping onto the crunchy coral pathway.

Then it was time to go: boarding the plane, waving from the windows, circling the glorious lagoon for one last time, then winging our way to the main island and closing that bitter-sweet tumultuous chapter of our lives –

Forever.

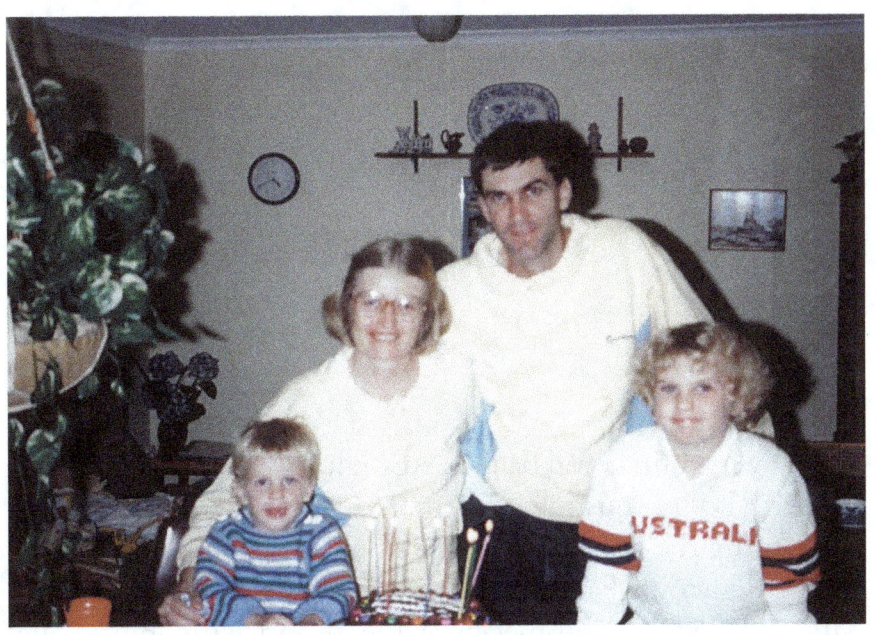

Our family at Wollongong following our return – November 1989.

Epilogue

Following our arrival back in Australia, we all went through a period of readjustment in our own very different ways.

During the few hours of our stop-over in Auckland on our return flight, we had a brief but treasured reconnection with Sam and Rachel, who met us at the airport with apples, hugs and tears. Their prayers, listening, and kindness all helped to soothe our heavy hearts, just as they had done so often in the past.

We then flew on to Sydney airport where our families welcomed us and, after fond reunions, we travelled to Mike's parents' place in Wollongong. Thomas climbed out of the car and ran down the garden path. Spotting a small fishpond along the way that contained a variety of goldfish, he shouted with considerable excitement: 'Quick Dad, get your'n speargun!'

Thomas had to adapt to innumerable changes in our western setting compared with the informal small-town lifestyle on Aitutaki. Not only were there dogs, crowds of *papa'as*, escalators, shopping trolleys and traffic lights, but the expectations in

Australia were literally worlds apart from everything he had ever known. I would sometimes turn around in Canberra shopping malls to find him peeing into an artificial pot plant: something that was perfectly acceptable in our previous life, except that on Aitutaki the shrubs were real.

Every day for months, he insisted on wearing his 'banana shorts' – a tiny red and blue pair so named because he'd worn them when fruit-picking on the island. They were already stained and torn, but gradually became scarcely recognisable at all, when the only remains were reduced to ragged ribbing. I finally hid them in a cupboard (in case he had a complete meltdown) and fobbed him off with other shorts until he eventually forgot about the originals and I could throw them out. It made sense for him to cling to anything familiar from his old life, since it was all he had ever known – and that included us as well. It seemed that the Velcro Boy had made a prolonged and intensive comeback...

Thirty years on, he has become a confident lawyer in charge of a legal team in the public service, and is now a committed husband and father of two gorgeous boys.

Rhiannon was glad to be back in Australia with family and friends, but from the time we returned, she denied that she could speak Māori at all. We found this very curious, since she had been so confidently bilingual before we left the island. Several months later, we had a visit from Tara, one of the OSB field officers, a planned follow-up to see how we were coping with the reverse culture shock that was common among returned volunteers. Tara was a New Zealand Maori herself, and during dinner at our place, we had explained our daughter's unexpected response. After the meal, she took Rhiannon to another room while we did the washing up, and she returned a short while later to report: 'She *does* still speak Māori.'

Apparently, when Tara had chatted to our daughter in her native tongue, Rhiannon had replied fluently in Māori. From this exchange, we presumed that she didn't want to attract unnecessary attention when mixing with other *papa'as* by using a language that she knew they didn't speak – so she'd responded by denying her skills altogether. Apart from that brief episode, no one ever heard her speak in Māori again.

Another important issue that we faced was whether or not to allow her to start Kindergarten with the next school year. Her birth-date in late April was close to the cut-off age for Canberra kids to begin school, and she had clearly had an unusual Preschool experience compared with her peers. However, with her habitual pragmatism, she insisted that she was ready to start in the January following our return, and did so with the unwavering determination that has characterised most of her life decisions ever since.

She has gone on to become an Emergency Medicine physician and Deputy Director of the Emergency Department of a large Australian hospital, who thrives on adrenaline and strong coffee.

As for Mike and me, we both went through a major time of upheaval in the months after our return. While it was good to have familiar people and places around us once again, we felt that we had undergone steep highs and lows during our two-year posting, whereas many others around us seemed to have journeyed through a mildly fluctuating continuum during the same period. The social disconnect was hard to bridge, and caused a disparate kind of isolation from the physical distance and cultural challenges that we had faced on Aitutaki. Many people skirted around discussions of our island life and the gaping heartache of my miscarriage. It seemed as though our experiences were uncomfortable and even embarrassing topics that they preferred to avoid, and conversations often skittered off into trivia and First World preoccupations.

If someone asked: 'How was your time away?' I learned to reply with a simple comment like: 'Challenging.' Most people were changing the subject by then or already walking away, so at least I hadn't wasted too much effort on trying to condense two years of intense experiences into one sentence. Very occasionally however, someone actually stopped and waited for a slightly longer answer; and even more rarely, they went on to converse with us for an hour or so. I vividly recall my sister weeping openly with me – one of the few who seemed to sense the depth of grief and lonely bewilderment that I still endured from our loss. Her tears were a precious gift to me.

Thankfully, however, I recovered well physically from my curette and we were delighted to conceive again shortly after our return. Chloe was born in September 1990, and was followed by Evan in 1994 – both very welcome additions to our family indeed. Chloe is now a committed primary school teacher, wife and mother of a gorgeous baby daughter; and Evan has recently completed his medical training and residency in Sydney.

When it came to day-to-day life back at home, we were sometimes surprised by the grumbling of our fellow Australians – it contrasted so starkly with the simple prospects and warm gratitude of the islanders. I remember standing in a large mall a few months after our return, surrounded by shops and shelves that were stacked with food, and hearing people complaining: 'It's so hard to decide what to have for dinner, isn't it?'

Really?

I remember thinking: 'You should try wondering what's for dinner when the supply ship hasn't been able to unload for three months and you're hoping someone will drop in a fish or some vegetables.'

And of course, even then our circumstances were so much better than many other folk on the planet – those who continue to struggle every single day for the most basic necessities of life.

Consequently, an enduring legacy of our posting has been to challenge any tendency I might have towards complacency or self-indulgence. If I sense myself degenerating into these habits, I see images of dirt-floored huts or children gnawing on taro, and they help me to realign my perspectives once again. In fact, we chose to take our four kids to India with a church working group in 2005 so that we could all get a good dose of 'How the rest of the world lives.' It has certainly served us well, although it's probably a good idea for all of us to go to a poor location every decade or so for a timely refresher course!

As regards our working life, just hearing the sound of a revving truck continued to cause both of us a sense of dread for many months after our return, and we were certainly glad to escape the onerous on-call demands and kitchen consultations of our island life. Despite this, it took us quite some time to settle back into work, and some of the hospital and general practice priorities felt trite and restrictive after the professional freedoms we had experienced on the island.

We have continued to benefit long term from learning to rely on clinical skills rather than expensive investigations in our work. The 'Rule of Thumb in Medicine' at the beginning of this book summarises what we'd learned during our posting, as well as the importance of developing realistic expectations about how effective our medical input was likely to be.

We have never returned to Aitutaki since our posting – something that many people find rather surprising. Perhaps it's due in part to the emotionally charged memories we have of that time, and especially our final months there. However, we also understand that the island has undergone many changes and become more tourist-orientated than previously, and we would prefer to remember the place and its people as they were when we lived there – the coinciding of their history and ours.

Although two years is a relatively short time-frame and easily lost in the span of a lifetime, our island experiences have had a major impact on our lives. With all the highs and lows that we encountered, we returned from the Cooks somewhat bruised and battered. The whole experience was much tougher than we had expected it would be. But it was important for us to acknowledge that we *had* made a difference too: the little ones safely delivered, the life-threatening conditions that responded to treatment, the medical input that ensured an improved quality of life, teaching local health workers further skills, and the opportunity to make the most of our difficulties and use our minimal resources to best effect. Of course, we learned a lot from the Māori too, about creativity, resilience, faith, gratitude and humour – all very valuable life lessons for us *papa'as* to emulate.

For all these things, we will remain forever grateful.

Would we recommend that others make a similar choice to have their own adventure? Our reply would be a qualified 'Yes' – so long as you're prepared to be changed and challenged in unexpected and powerful ways – sure, it's the adventure of a lifetime…

When all is said and done, we've never regretted the decision to go, and have grown in ways that we'd never have anticipated otherwise.

As Michael once commented: 'Possibly there's a little bit of Polynesian within each one of us' – and maybe, it's just hibernating inside of us until we're let loose on a tiny atoll, where it can burst out and work its islander charm on even the most restrained and unlikely of *papa'as!*

Christmas Card from Dr Rua 28th December, 1989.

Dr Mike and Michele Browne and family,
I remember you all with affection. Thank you very much "imo pectore" for the valuable services and ready assistance rendered to the people of Aitutaki. I consider Aitutaki a lucky island. Your contributions (both) and sacrifices will remain as one difficult to forget or substitute.
Within the 40 years of my service, you both are one of the few I find real pleasure and pride in working with. I thank you both for considering Aitutaki as a place to work, although it is a tiny place compared to your previous experiences.
May God pave the way for success in your future careers.
I pray all are well with you and the family this Christmas and New Year, and that the joy and peace that come your way remain unceasingly.
"Kia orana."
God bless.
Dr Rua.
28/12/1989.

A Note from the Author

Did you enjoy my book?

If so, I would be very grateful if you could write a review and publish it at your point of purchase. Your review, even a brief one, will help other readers to decide whether or not they'll enjoy my work.

Do you want to be notified of new releases?

If so, please **sign up to the AIA Publishing email list**. You'll find the sign-up button on the right-hand side under the photo at **www.aiapublishing.com**. Of course, your information will never be shared, and the publisher won't inundate you with emails, just let you know of new releases.

About the Author

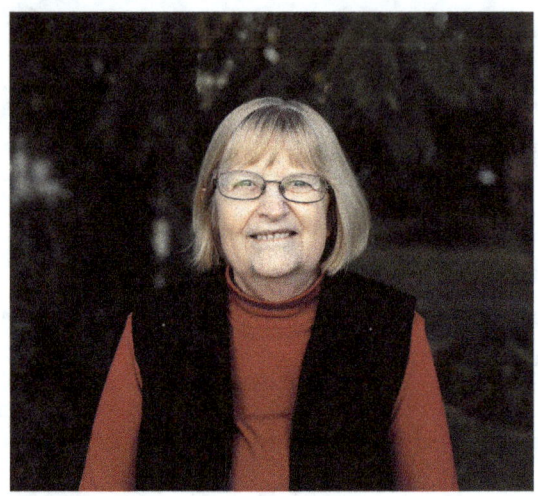

Michele is a doctor, wife, mother, grandmother and mentor. She has worked in general medical practice for four decades, since graduating in Medicine at the University of New South Wales (Sydney, Australia) in 1981. Following this, she and her husband Michael (also a GP) lived and worked in Canberra and, more recently, in the beautiful Shoalhaven region, where they currently work in a large group practice.

'Beyond the Reef' is her first book, a memoir of the two-year volunteer service that Michele and Michael completed in 1988-89 while accompanied by their two very young children.

Glossary of Māori Terms.

Akama – shame, embarrassment, fear of being ridiculed or censured.
Amuri – village on Aitutaki.
Are-nikau – thatched **Pandanus** palm-leaf shelter.
Arutanga – village on Aitutaki.
Atoll – island formed by a largely underwater pre-historic volcano surrounded by a coral reef that creates an enclosed lagoon.
Cocophone – ukulele made from an empty halved coconut-shell.
Eis – flower garlands. (Cook Island Māori has no 'L' so Polynesian 'leis' are called 'eis'.)
Frangipani – see **Tipani**.
Ika – multiple meanings: 'fish', 'ocean' or 'vagina'.
Iti – small.
Ivi – bone.
Kaikai – 'eat, eat' or feast.
Kaivi – a hard-shelled tropical fruit with edible seeds that resembled almonds.
Kapu – cup.
Kata – laugh.
Kete – basket.
Ki – full.
Kia orana – a Māori greeting meaning "Live on!" or "Be blessed!"
Kiri – skin. (Also used as a derisive term for the 'foreskin' of uncircumcised boys.)
Kopu – stomach.

Kumara – sweet potato(es).
Kuru – Breadfruit – large, round, green-skinned fruits containing dense white pulp.
Mamas – the term Māori used for mothers or older women.
Marae – islander sacred areas or constructions.
Maru – gentle.
Mata – dimples in coconuts that can be pierced to access coconut milk inside.
Mito – a **Surgeonfish** – a reef fish with scalpel-like spines near their tales, equivalent to the sharpness of a No. 15 scalpel blade.
Moko – gecko or small lizard, often living indoors, that feeds on insects, spiders, etc.
Motu – small, usually uninhabited, islet within the lagoon, often used for day-trips or fishing.
Motus in Aitutaki Lagoon – *Akitua* (on which the resort was located), *Angarei, Niura, Mangere, Papau, Tavaerua iti, Tavaerua nui, Akaiami* (which had a private house on it), *Muritapua, Tekopua, Tapuaetai* (One Foot Island), *Motukitiu, Moturakau, Rapota, Maina* – clockwise around lagoon.
Nikaupara – village on Aitutaki.
Northern Group Islands of the Cook Islands: Nassau, Palmerston, Penrhyn (Tongareva), Manihiki, Rakahanga, Pukapuka, Suwarrow.
Nu – green coconuts containing refreshing liquid.
Oatu – to give away.
Okaru – orange-brown semi-mature coconuts that contain coconut cream.
Padua – mother-of-pearl from trochus shells, used in jewellery and decorations.
Pandanus – wide-leaved short palm trees.
Papas – the term Māori used for fathers or older men.
Papa'as – non-Māori people.
Pareu – rectangular cloth used as a wrap-around garment.
Pawpaws – large soft tropical fruits, usually yellow or orange in

colour when ripe.
Pepe – baby.
Pipi – shellfish.
Pok'e – pudding made from mashed bananas and arrowroot paste, cooked in an **Umu.**
Poro - ball.
Reureu – village on Aitutaki.
Rima – hand, five.
Rua – two.
Rukau – a bush with edible leaves that resembled baby spinach.
Southern Group Islands of the Cook Islands: Rarotonga, Mangaia, Atiu, Aitutaki, Mauke, Mitiaro, Manuae, Takutea.
Taku – mine.
Tiare – flower.
Tiare Maori – Gardenias, fragrant white flowers.
Tipani – Frangipani – trees growing fragrant white and pink or yellow flowers.
Toru – three.
Toto – blood.
Trevally – moderate sized silvery edible tropical fish.
Tua – story.
Tuatua – talk.
Tuka – sugar.
Tutaka – the regular inspection of dwellings/properties throughout the island.
Umu – Māori ground ovens for producing **Kaikai** food. See also **Umukais.**
Umukais – Māori ground ovens for producing **Kaikai** food. See also **Umu.**
Ureia – village on Aitutaki.
Uto – mature brown coconuts containing hard nut for eating/shredding.
Vaipae – village on Aitutaki.
Vaipeka – village on Aitutaki.

Glossary of Medical and Other Terms.

Abscess – swollen red collection of **Pus** in a localised infection.
Acute – sudden onset, or short-term, that is, less than 3 months.
Adrenaline – hormone (natural or synthetic): constricts blood vessels and stimulates heart.
Afebrile – normal temperature, no fever.
AIDS – Acquired Immunodeficiency Syndrome – loss of the body's immunity due to **HIV** infection.
Air-bagging – hand compression of rubber bag attached to endotracheal tube or face mask.
Air travel when pregnant – Most airlines didn't allow women pregnant beyond 28wks to fly.
Allergens – factors that stimulate allergic reactions, e.g. foods, inhaled agents, etc.
Amoxicillin – a broad-spectrum **Penicillin**-based **Antibiotic**.
Amniotic fluid – fluid surrounding the **Foetus** in the **Uterus**. See also **Liquor**.
Anaesthetic – medication to induce generalised sleep (**General Anaesthetic**) or localised tissue numbness (**Local Anaesthetic**).
Analgesic – medication to relieve pain, e.g. **Paracetamol**, **Morphine**.
Ante-natal – timeframe before birth; pregnancy-related.

Antibiotic – medication that immobilises or kills **Bacteria** (oral or injected).
Anti-epileptic – medication to treat or reverse **Seizures** or **Epileptic Fits**.
Anti-hypertensive – agent used to lower **Blood pressure (BP)**.
Anti-nauseant – medication (oral or injected) to treat nausea and/or vomiting.
Arterial spasm – intense contractions of artery, limiting blood supply to local tissue.
Aspirate – (noun) – substance(s) drawn from organs or body cavities.
Aspirated – (verb) – inhaled substances in airways, lungs or nasal passages.
Atoll – island formed by a largely underwater pre-historic volcano surrounded by a coral reef that creates an enclosed lagoon.
Atopic – familial tendency to develop hay fever and/or eczema and/or asthma.
AUD – Australian Dollars. Approximate exchange rate in 1988-89 was 1.30 **NZD**:1.00 **AUD**.
Australia Day – 26th January annually – marks the arrival of the British First Fleet that began the European colonisation of Australia on 26/1/1788.
Australian Volunteers Abroad – **AVA** – later renamed as the **OSB** – **Overseas Services Bureau**: a non-government aid organisation that connected Australian professionals with overseas requests for assistance.
AVA – see **Australian Volunteers Abroad**.
AWOL – Absent Without Leave; disappeared.
Axillae – underarms.
Bacterial – infection by bacteria – usually responsive to **Antibiotics**.
Bacterial meningitis – **Bacterial** infection of **Meninges** (tissue layers surrounding the brain).
Bactrim – a sulphonamide broad-spectrum **Antibiotic** (tablet or

syrup).

Balls – colloquial term for testicles.

Barotrauma – trauma caused by sudden changes in air pressure affecting enclosed cavities, e.g. lungs, sinuses, middle ear.

Bearing down – active urge to push in **Labour,** usually once the **Cervix** is fully **dilated** (10cm).

Bends – common term for decompression sickness where bubbles of nitrogen in the blood expand with rapid air pressure changes causing damage to surrounding tissues, e.g. stroke.

Birth canal – vagina.

Black Dwell-cath – a large bore **Cannula** used for rapid movement of fluids into or out of the body.

Blighted ovum – fertilised **Ovum** (female egg cell) which fails to differentiate into **Foetus** and **Placenta,** leading to a non-viable pregnancy and usually an **Inevitable Miscarriage**.

Blood Glucose Levels (BGL) – See **Blood Sugar Levels.**

Blood Pressure – **BP** – measurement of pressure within the body's arterial system.

Blood Sugar Levels – **BSL** – measurement of sugar (glucose) levels in blood; commonly range from 3 – 11mmol/litre in non-diabetics. Sometimes called **Blood Glucose Levels (BGL).**

Bodily fluids – bodily secretions, e.g. blood, saliva, urine, breastmilk, genital, **Pus**, etc.

Body Mass Index – weight of person in kg divided by height in metres squared (kg/m²).

Bonney's dissecting forceps – small surgical forceps used in minor surgical procedures.

Box – genital protection device for use by males when batting in cricket.

BP – abbreviation for **Blood Pressure.**

Brachial nerve block – shoulder region injection of **Local Anaesthetic** to numb arm/hand.

Breech – **Foetal position** where **Foetus**'s buttocks or lower limbs are the **Presenting parts**.
Bronchiolitis – infection or inflammation of bronchioles (small airways).
Bronchitis – infection or inflammation of the bronchi (larger airways).
BSL – see **Blood Sugar Levels**.
Burley – food/bait to attract fish when fishing.
Butt – colloquial term for bottom or **Buttock**.
Butterfly Cannula – small **Cannula** for insertion into blood vessels.
Buttock – bottom or **Butt**.
Caesarean – surgery to deliver a **Foetus** through incised abdominal wall opening.
Cannula – **Intravenous** needle situated in vein to insert fluids, blood and/or medications, or to withdraw blood.
Carbs/ Carbohydrate – plant-based sugars.
Cardiac arrest – cessation of heart action.
Carrier rate – percentage of population infected with a specific pathogen.
Central Nervous System – **CNS** – made up of the brain and spinal cord.
Cerebrospinal fluid – **CSF** – fluid surrounding the brain and spinal cord.
Cerebrospinal pressures – pressures within the **CSF** around the spinal cord and brain.
Cervix/Cervical – the **Uterine** opening.
Chest cavity – space within the rib cage.
Chromic catgut – a suture material. 2/0, 3/0 = thickness of suture (smaller the number = greater the thickness).
Chronic – longer term, that is greater than 3-6 months duration.
Circa – originating around the period of a certain date.
Circumcision – surgical removal of foreskin of penis.

Clinically – assessment using only history and examination, not imaging/pathology testing.
CNS – see **Central Nervous System**.
Conjunctivae – delicate tissues overlying surface of eyes and under eyelids.
Conjunctivitis – infection or inflammation of **Conjunctivae**.
Contagious – high likelihood of spread of infection.
Convulsion – see **Fit** or **Grand mal** seizure.
CSF – **Cerebrospinal fluid** – fluid surrounding the brain and spinal cord.
Curettage/Curette – see **D&C**.
Cyanosis – blue skin colour due to low oxygen levels in arterial blood.
D&C – **Dilatation and Curettage** – surgical **Dilatation** of **Cervix** using metal instruments and scraping (**Curettage**) to remove **Uterine** contents.
Debrided – cutting away damaged flesh and/or foreign material to clean up a wound.
Degloving injury – peeled off flesh, tendons, nerves and/or blood vessels.
Dehydration – net loss of fluid from the body due to imbalance of fluid intake and output.
Delivery – process of giving birth to baby, either vaginally of via **Caesarean**. See also **Labour**.
Diagnosis – name of disorder or medical condition causing a patient's **Symptoms**/disease.
Dilated/Dilatation – (degree of) opening e.g. **Cervix**, eye pupil, etc.
Diuretic – medication to remove excess fluid from body and/or decrease **Blood pressure**.
DIY – abbreviation for Do-It-Yourself, i.e. homemade.
Do a runner – run away, escape.
Drop-off – outer edge of reef that followed the side of the **Atoll**-forming volcanic mountain down into the sea.

Duodenum – first part of the small bowel adjacent to the stomach.
Dwell-cath – a large bore **Cannula** used for rapidly inserting or removing fluids into/out of the body.
Eardrum – **Tympanic membrane** – membrane that separates the ear canal from **Middle Ear**. When red and/or swollen, it can indicate a **Middle ear infection**.
Elective Caesarean – pre-arranged **Caesarean** prior to spontaneous **Labour** commencing.
Elixir – liquid medication, e.g. cough syrup.
Emergency Caesarean – urgent **Caesarean**, often due to **Foetal distress**.
Encephalitis – infection/inflammation of brain tissue.
Endocarditis – infection/inflammation of heart valves and/or heart muscle.
Endotracheal tube – small rubber tube inserted through **Vocal cords** to control upper airways.
Envenomation – bite by organisms which inject venom, such as spiders or snakes.
Epileptic – person who has **Seizures** or **Convulsions**. See **Grand Mal Fit**.
Episiotomy – surgical cut into vaginal opening (**Perineum**) to facilitate **Delivery** of infant.
Established labour – when labour is consistently progressing towards **Delivery**.
Ether – an inhaled form of **General Anaesthetic** agent to induce sleep.
Expired – out of date; can also mean 'died.'
Exudate – biological fluid secreted from skin, body cavities, organs or organism. See also **Aspirate** and **Bodily fluids.**
Face presentation – where **Foetal** face is the **Presenting part** during **Labour**.
Failure to progress – When **Labour** stalls and the **Foetus** is not

being delivered.
Febrile convulsion – **Grand mal seizure** or **Fit** caused by a high fever.
Fit – Convulsion – uncontrolled nerve messages across **CNS**, causing erratic muscle movements and/or altered mental function/level of consciousness. See **Grand mal seizure**.
Foetal/Foetus – developing infant in the **Uterus**.
Foetal distress – where the **Foetus**'s heart rate falls during **Labour** suggesting that the blood supply to **Foetal** organs is inadequate.
Footling breech – **Breech** where **Presenting parts** are **Foetal** knee/s and/or foot/feet.
Frangipani – trees growing fragrant white, yellow or pink flowers. Called **Tipani** in Māori.
Frontal Sinuses – bilateral **Sinuses** in the centre of the forehead.
Full term – the end of pregnancy (about 40 weeks' **Gestation**) from first day of the last period.
Fully Dilated – maximally **Dilated** or opened up, e.g. when **Cervix** is 10cm wide.
Functional obstruction – bowel obstruction caused by impaired **Peristalsis** rather than a physical blockage. See **Ileus** also.
Gastro/Gastroenteritis – **Bacterial, Viral** or Parasitic infection of the gut, causing bowel wall inflammation and nausea and/or vomiting and/or diarrhoea.
General Anaesthetic – **Anaesthetic** medication to induce generalised sleep.
General Practitioner – **GP** or Family physician – doctor providing **Primary care**.
Gestation – length of pregnancy. See **Full term** also.
Gestational diabetes – diabetes (high **Blood Sugar Levels**) during pregnancy.
Giving-set – tube and connections that attach **IV** (**Intravenous**) fluid bags to **Cannula**.

Gluteal region – buttocks, **Butt**.
GP – see **General Practitioner**.
Grand mal seizure – **Convulsion** affecting the whole body. See **Fit**.
Grand multiparas – women who have had at least five previous pregnancies of more than 26 weeks' **Gestation**.
Greenlane – a hospital in Auckland, New Zealand that included a paediatric unit.
Gumboots – rubber boots used for gardening or outdoor activities.
Haemoglobin – iron carrier in red blood cells (normal range is approx. 115 – 160g/litre).
Haemorrhage – heavy (possibly life-threatening) bleeding.
Haemorrhagic Disease of the Newborn – postnatal bleeding in a newborn due to Vitamin K deficiency.
Haemorrhagic Form of Dengue Fever – mosquito-borne infection causing bleeding within body organs and potentially multiple **Organ failure**.
Haemorrhoidectomy – resection of **Haemorrhoids** or **Piles**.
Haemorrhoids – varicose veins in the anal and/or rectal regions, also known as **Piles**.
Head-colds – common term for **Upper respiratory illnesses**.
Heavy Nupicaine – long-obsolete **Local Anaesthetic** agent mixed with a dense glucose solution and inserted into **Spinal canal** of seated patient so that it sinks to the lowest parts of the canal and anaesthetises **Saddle region**. Used for **Obstetrics** and pelvic surgery.
HIV – see **Human Immunodeficiency Virus**.
Humidicribs – enclosed hospital crib providing constant temperature.
Hypertension – high **Blood pressure** (**BP**), damages heart and blood vessels.
Ileus – bowel obstruction caused by impaired **Peristalsis**. See also **Functional obstruction**.
Impetigo – **Bacterial** skin infection characterised by scabs, blisters, redness and **Pus**.

Inevitable Miscarriage – **Miscarriage** that spontaneously proceeds from threatened to irreversible **Miscarriage.**
In situ – in position.
In utero – in the womb.
Intra-abdominal – within the abdomen.
Intracranial pressure – pressure inside the skull affecting brain position and function.
Intramuscular – within the muscle layers.
Intrauterine – within the **Uterus** or womb.
Intravenous – **IV** – within vein; fluids or medications inserted via **Cannula** into vein.
Intubation – **Endotracheal** rubber tube inserted through **Vocal cords** into upper airways.
Intussusception – condition where bowel wall inverts internally causing bowel obstruction.
Irregular contractions – not fully **Established labour**, erratic **Uterine** contractions.
IV – see **Intravenous**.
Ketamine – an injected **General Anaesthetic** medication.
Kidney dish – a kidney-shaped metal or plastic bowl to hold small medical/surgical items.
Kiwi – colloquial term for New Zealanders. Also: a flightless bird found in New Zealand.
Labour – process of regular **Uterine** contractions to dilate **Cervix** and expel **Foetus (Delivery).**
Laparotomy – abdominal surgery to explore and treat **Intra-abdominal** pathology.
Laryngeal region/Larynx – largest airway at commencement of bronchial system, includes **Vocal cords**.
Laryngoscope – torch with curved blade for visualising the **Vocal cords**, throat and **Larynx**.
Lax – flabby, lacking in muscle tone or elasticity.

Lino/Linoleum – a form of vinyl floor covering.
Liquor – alcoholic drinks. Also: **Amniotic fluid** in the womb surrounding a **Foetus**.
Local Anaesthetic – **Anaesthetic** agent that numbs a localised area of skin/tissue.
Long-drops – primitive toilets – deep hole in the ground with a shelf at the top to sit on.
Loo – colloquial term for toilet.
Lumbar puncture – insertion of sterile needle into **Spinal canal** to measure **Cerebrospinal pressures**, and/or remove **Cerebrospinal fluid (CSF)** to test for blood, cells and/or organisms.
Lumbar vertebrae – lowest five **Vertebrae** in the spine/spinal column.
Lymphangitis – infection causing red streaking along a limb towards the local lymph nodes.
Malignancy – cancer.
Mastitis – infection of the breast, usually associated with breastfeeding.
Mauriceau–Smellie–Veit manoeuvre – Method of delivering a breech: after trunk and legs are delivered, the **Foetal** head is rotated to face the mother's back, then the operator's left hand is inserted into the mother's vagina, and a finger placed into the **Foetal** mouth to flex the neck. Traction then applied by the operator's right hand to the infant's shoulder while easing out the baby's head.
Meninges – delicate tissue layers surrounding the brain and spinal cord.
Meningitis – infection or inflammation of **Meninges** – can be **Viral** or **Bacterial.**
Middle ear – section of ear between the **Eardrum** and the Inner ear.
Middle ear infection – infection behind the **Eardrum** (**Tympanic membrane**), often causing **Eardrum** to be red and/or bulging.
Milo – a powdered chocolate milk drink.
Miscarriage – spontaneous loss of pregnancy.
Monaural otoscope – an old-fashioned wooden horn for listening to

Foetal heartbeats during pregnancy and/or **Labour**.
Morphine – opiate-based **Analgesic** medication, can be oral or injected.
Multip/Multiparous – a woman who has had at least one prior pregnancy beyond 26 weeks' gestation.
Nappies – diapers, composed of cloth (for us), but commonly now disposable.
Nappy-bags – carrier bags for **Nappies** (diapers) and baby paraphernalia.
Naso-gastric tube – tube inserted through nose into stomach to withdraw gastric contents and/or insert fluids or medications.
NAUI – the National Association of Underwater Instructors, begun in the USA in 1960.
Nerdy – colloquial term for a socially awkward but often academically capable person.
Neurological – nerve or nervous system related.
Neville-Barnes forceps – large metal forceps for delivery of a **Foetal** head during **Labour**.
NZD – New Zealand Dollars. Approximate exchange rate in 1988-9 was 1.30**NZD**:1.00**AUD**.
Obstetrics – practice of caring for and delivering both pregnant patients and their babies.
Occipital position – where the back of the **Foetal** head is the **Presenting part** in **Obstetrics**.
Occiput – back of the head. See **Occipital position**.
Occult – 'hidden'; relates to 'black magic' or witchcraft.
Ophthalmologist – eye surgeon.
Organ failure – loss of function of major body organ/system, e.g. cardiac/respiratory/renal failure.
Oro-pharynx – the mouth and back of the throat (**Pharynx**).
OSB – Overseas Services Bureau – an Australian non-government aid organisation previously known as **Australian Volunteers Abroad**

(**AVA**).
Ovum – the female germ cell or 'egg' which, after fertilisation, can develop into a **Foetus**.
Oxytocin – hormone which stimulates **Uterine** contractions and ejection of breast milk. Chemically identical with **Syntocinon**.
Pap smear – abbreviation for Papanicolaou smear – scraping of surface cells of **Cervix** to check for possible abnormalities including **Cervical** cancer.
Paracetamol – medication (tablets or syrup) to control fever and pain (**Analgesic**).
Penicillin – well known **Antibiotic**.
Perforating injury – piercing of skin and/or underlying tissue by a foreign body.
Perineum – vulva; vaginal or **Birth canal** opening.
Peristalsis – regular contractions of intestinal wall, to propel bowel contents forward.
Peritoneal lavage – running **Saline** into **Intra-abdominal** cavity through a **Giving set** and **Dwell-cath**, then lowering **Giving set** so that blood/contaminants in cavity can drain out.
Pharynx – back of the throat.
Piles – colloquial term for **Haemorrhoids**.
Placenta – **Intrauterine** organ in pregnancy which allows transfer of oxygen, nutrition and waste products to and from the **Foetus**.
Plasma – **Intravenous** fluid containing electrolytes (sodium, potassium, etc) and proteins. Also: fluid component of blood that transports electrolytes, blood cells, hormones, etc.
Plaster – white bandages infiltrated with powder that sets after water is added – used to immobilise fractures.
Play-doh – non-edible dough for child's play – either homemade or commercially produced.
Post-natal – time-frame following birth.
Post-op/Post-operative – time-frame following surgery.

Post-partum haemorrhage – heavy vaginal bleeding following **Delivery** of an infant.
Presenting part – **Foetal** body part adjacent to **Cervix** and/or **Birth canal**.
Primary care – medical care for unscreened or self-referred patients.
Primip/Primiparous – first pregnancy.
Provisional diagnosis – initial **Diagnosis** that probably explains the presenting **Symptoms**.
Pulmonary – pertaining to the lungs.
Pus – foul-smelling discoloured fluid in infections and **Abscesses**.
PVC – polyvinyl chloride – strong but lightweight plastic used for plumbing pipes, etc.
Rehydration – increased oral or **IV** fluids given to treat **Dehydration**.
Respiratory arrest – cessation of breathing.
Rheumatic Heart Disease – damage to heart valves by Streptococcus **Bacteria**.
Ring block – **Local Anaesthetic** inserted around base of an appendage, e.g. finger, penis, etc.
Royal Australian College of General Practitioners (RACGP) – the only Australian postgraduate college in the 1980s that provided specialist training for **General Practitioners** (**GP**s). There is now a second college called ACRRM – the Australian College of Rural and Remote Medicine.
Saddle block – a spinal block causing numbness to the **Saddle region**.
Saddle region – anatomical region including **Perineum**, **Buttocks** and inner thighs.
Saline – sterile **Intravenous** fluid containing sodium chloride in the same dilution as **Plasma**.
Scalpel – sharp-bladed surgical instrument for incising tissue.
Secondary organ failure – loss of major organ function due to serious illness/infection.
Seizure – see **Fit, Convulsion** or **Grand Mal Fit**.

Septic arthritis – infection (usually **Bacterial**) within a joint.
Sinuses – aeration spaces of facial bones to assist with lightening the skull and humidifying the airways.
Sluice room – room for washing and sterilising medical equipment.
Solution B – a chemical agent used in the hand-developing of X-rays.
Sonicaid – a portable ultrasound machine to check for **Foetal** heart sounds.
Sphygmomanometer – **Blood pressure (BP)** measuring device.
Spinal block – **Local Anaesthetic** inserted into **Spinal canal** to numb adjacent region.
Spinal canal – area enclosing the spinal cord that contains **Cerebrospinal fluid (CSF).**
Steroids – medications used to suppress inflammation and/or reduce swelling.
Stroke – brain damage due to disrupted blood supply to a region of the brain.
Suction device – suction tube attached to pump to extract fluid from mouth, airways, or body cavities.
Surgeonfish – reef fish with scalpel-like spines near the tale, equivalent to the sharpness of a No. 15 scalpel blade. Known as *Mito* in Māori.
Symptoms – features of illness that are detectable or a patient is aware of, e.g. pain, fever.
Syntocinon – injectable synthetic **Oxytocin**, used to limit **Post-natal Uterine** bleeding.
Testosterone – male sex hormone.
Third World – term used in the 1980s that now denotes Developing Nations.
Titration – measurement or mixture of chemical substance/s.
Topical – medication applied to skin or mucous membranes.
Tourniquet – tight band applied to a limb to temporarily cut off the blood flow.
Transducer gel – liquid used to transmit sound waves into audible

(**Sonicaid**) or visual (**Ultrasound**) forms.
Tympanic membrane – see **Eardrum.**
Ultrasound – medical device using sound waves to create visual images.
Undiagnosed – not previously diagnosed, no medical awareness of a relevant condition.
Uni – short for University.
Upper respiratory illnesses – 'common cold', **Head-cold,** infections in upper airways, etc.
Urinary catheter – bladder tube to drain and measure urine output.
Ute – utility van: open-backed truck with enclosed cabin, used as ambulance on Aitutaki.
Uterus/Uterine – womb.
Vaginal examination – insertion of gloved digits to assess vagina, **Cervix** or pelvic organs.
Venepuncture – insertion of needle or **Cannula** into vein to insert blood, medications, fluids, etc. or remove blood. See **Intravenous** also.
Vernix – white cheesy substance that may coat the **Foetal** skin to protect it **In utero.**
Vertebrae – bones making up the spine.
Vertex presentation – **Foetal** head as the **Presenting part**, as in normal **Labour.**
VIPs – abbreviation for 'Very Important People.'
Viral/Virus – simple (usually single-celled) organism that can infect a host organism.
Viral meningitis – **Viral** infection of **Meninges**, doesn't respond to **Antibiotics.**
Viral upper respiratory illnesses – **Viral** infections in upper airways. See **Upper respiratory illnesses.**
Vitals – checks of blood pressure, pulse/breathing rates, temperature, etc.

Vocal cords – two adjacent membranes in **Larynx** that vibrate to allow speech/sounds.

Weetbix – a wheat-based breakfast cereal.

Wheeze – whistling noise when breathing, due to constricted airways, as in asthma.

Yachties – sailing enthusiasts.

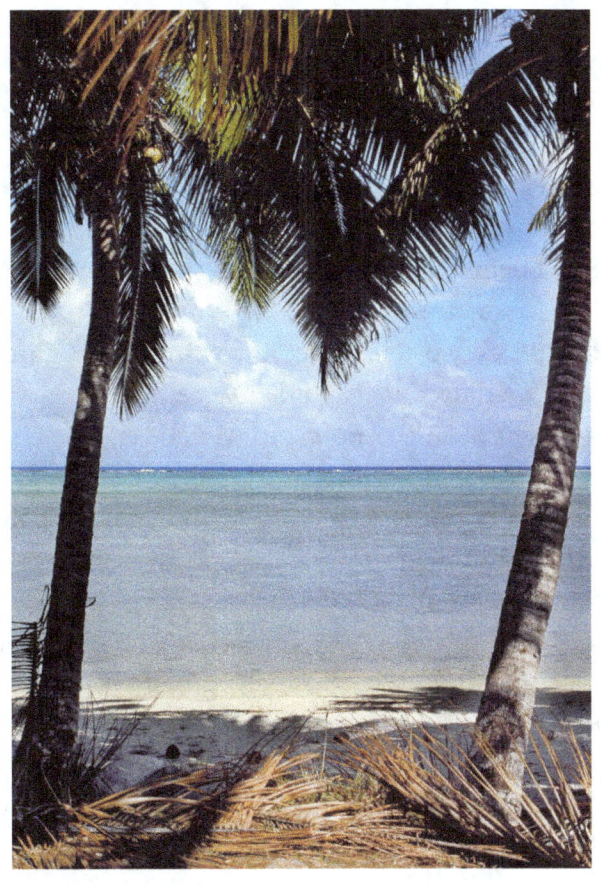

Beach view from Silcock's Beach towards the lagoon.

Timeline of Aitutaki Posting.

August, 1987 – Interview with OSB in Canberra.

Dec, 1987 – Car (Hilda) packed and sent to Sydney - Auckland - Rarotonga - Aitutaki.

13/1/1988 – Flight (10.30 a.m.) Canberra to Melbourne for initial one-week briefing.

21/1/1988 – Flight (4 p.m.) Melbourne - Auckland - Rarotonga - arrived 5.30 a.m. on same date.

21/1 - 5/2/1988 – Two-week in-country briefing in Rarotonga. The car arrives and we moved it to another vessel.

6/2/1988 – Flight from Rarotonga to Aitutaki.

12/2/1988 – Car (Hilda) arrives in Aitutaki.

3/1988 – Mike's parents (Mac & Ena Browne) visit for 3 weeks. 3-day trip to Akaiami with Bonita, Mac & Ena.

28/4/1988 – Rhiannon's 3rd birthday.

4/1988 – Michele commences Women's Clinic on Monday afternoons.

25/5/1988 – Thomas's 1st birthday.

27/6 - 8/7/1988 – 2 weeks of Anaesthetics in Rarotonga.

3/7 - 16/7/1988 – Appels' visit for 2 weeks (Raro for 5 days, Aitutaki for 9 days.)

Late 8/1988 – Sonicaid arrives at Aitutaki.

9/1988 – Michele's parents (Bruce & Marguerite Cole) visit for 2 weeks.

10/1988 – 1-week of annual leave on Akaiami with Bonita.
11/1988 – Michele begins working two half-days per week regularly.
11/1988 – Mark & Karl visit and do scuba diving course with Mike.
1/1989 – 1-week trip to Akaiami with volunteer family (from Mauke) and Bonita.
1/1989 – Bonita leaves Aitutaki for NZ & Australia before returning to the USA.
11/3/89 - 5/5/1989 – Mike's parents (Mac & Ena Browne) return for 8 weeks.
23 - 26/3/1989 – Michele does the scuba course with Father Luke.
2/1989 – Rhiannon starts Preschool 3 mornings per week.
4/1989 – Sam and Rachel Stephens arrive in Aitutaki for 4 months.
28/4/1989 – Rhiannon's 4th birthday.
5/1989 – Vandermoezels visit for 2 weeks. Randles visit for 1 week.
25/5/1989 – Thomas's 2nd birthday.
6/2089 – Mike and I begin working alternate weeks full-time. (Davises visit for 2 weeks.)
6/1989 – Rhiannon starts Preschool 5 mornings per week.
7/1989 – Hingleys visit for 4 weeks.
16/8/1989 – Stephens leave Aitutaki.
8/1989 – 1-week annual leave – we stay at Silcock's Beach cottage.
8/1989 – Ewan's family visit from the UK.
9/1989 – Michele's Sister: Marguerite & husband Philip Jones & 4 kids: Heidi, Ben, Sarah & Bronwyn/Mother: Marguerite Cole/ Friend: Megan Hawkins – all visit us for 2 weeks.
10/1989 – Felix Muggli visits for 2 weeks.
29/10/1989 – D&C.
6/11/1989 – Our flight Aitutaki - Rarotonga.
9/11/1989 – Flight Rarotonga - Auckland (seeing Stephens at airport) - Sydney.
10/11/1989 – Arrival Sydney airport.

www.ingramcontent.com/pod-product-compliance
Lightning Source LLC
Chambersburg PA
CBHW071556080526
44588CB00010B/929